REDHOTTOUCH

JAIYA AND JON HANAUER

with Julie Jeffries

REDHOTTOUCH

A HEAD-TO-TOE HANDBOOK FOR
MIND-BLOWING ORGASMS

THREE RIVERS PRESS
NEW YORK

Published in the United States by Three Rivers Press, an imprint of the Crown Publishing
Group, a division of Random House, Inc., New York.

www.crownpublishing.com

Originally published in the United States by Broadway Books, an imprint of the Crown
Publishing Group, a division of Random House, Inc., New York, in 2008.

THREE RIVERS PRESS and the Tugboat design are registered trademarks of Random House, Inc.

Illustrations by Brett Johnson

Book design by Casey Hampton

LIBRARY OF CONGRESS CATALOGING-IN-PUBLICATION DATA
Hanauer, Jaiya.
Red hot touch : a head-to-toe handbook for mind-blowing orgasms / by Jaiya and
Jon Hanauer with Julie Jeffries ; illustrations by Brett Johnson.—1st ed.
p. cm.
1. Sex instruction—Popular works.   2. Sex—Popular works.   3. Man-woman
relationships.   I. Hanauer, Jon.   II. Jeffries, Julie.   III. Title.
HQ31.H3374   2008
613.9'6—dc22   2007036836

ISBN 978-0-7679-2821-2

PRINTED IN THE UNITED STATES OF AMERICA

7 9 10 8

The human hand is so beautifully formed, its actions are so powerful, so free and yet so delicate that there is no thought of its complexity as an instrument; we use it as we draw our breath, unconsciously.

—SIR CHARLES BELL, *The Hand, Its Mechanism and Vital Endowments, As Evincing Design* (1840)

CONTENTS

REDHOTTOUCH

THE FUTURE IS IN YOUR HANDS

If you were asked which part of your body was your most powerful asset in bed, how would you answer—after you stopped blushing, of course? Maybe you'd admit that your tongue knows some pretty tantalizing tricks, or deem your derrière as your most attention-getting gift. Who knows, maybe your beautifully groomed, extraordinarily endowed privates never fail to impress. Whatever your response, we'll bet we know of one area of your anatomy that wouldn't immediately cross your mind: your hands. Sure, hands may be essential for undoing buttons, unzipping zippers, and occasionally squeezing the goods, but beyond that, what do your hands truly have to offer?

Well, allow us to fill you in.

Hands are the most nimble instruments on the human body. They can do all sorts of amazing things, from playing a soul-stirring piano concerto to performing open-heart surgery. Without hands, the Sistine Chapel would have never been painted. The statue of David? Just a ho-hum hunk of marble. And you could forget about cheering on Roger Clemens as he strikes out another batter with his incredible fastball. Given all the things our hands have accomplished and still do to this day, they should be pulling off some equally dazzling feats of dexterity *in* bed as well as out.

And yet, for some reason, once we lay our hands on each other, it's as if we devolve millions of years, resorting to moves that are almost Cro-Magnon in their simplicity. We grab, we grope, we paw our way around. If we're lucky enough to get ahold of someone's privates, we oafishly pump up and down like we're on a pogo stick, or (if it's a woman) wiggle our finger a little. That's hardly what we'd call sophisticated, and it's a crying shame, since in terms of *potential,* hands can do much, much more. Limiting ourselves in this way is like seeing Albert Einstein work as an accountant, or Pavarotti deejay karaoke parties. Contrary to popular opinion, your hands can—and should— provide amazing, earth-moving, angels-singing experiences . . . that is, if anyone knew what to do with them.

That's where we come in.

As certified sexological bodyworkers, we've been trained to teach people how to rub each other the right way from head to toe and everywhere in between. Genital massage encompasses a large part of our curriculum, and our students are always surprised (and happy!) to find out that there are more than fifty ways to stroke, squeeze, and please someone south of the border. Throw in the techniques we teach students on how to stimulate other areas of the anatomy from the earlobes to the toes, and all told, our students come away with more than 150 new manual moves, from Little Earthquake (which creates great below-the-belt buzz) to the Twist 'n' Shout (so named because it will have him hollering for more).

If you had no idea that your hands could make the human body hit a high note in so many ways, that's only because you're not used to seeing your hands as the virtuosos they truly are. To help open your eyes to all the pleasurable possibilities that are within your grasp, here are a few things to keep in mind.

HANDY FACT #1: YOUR HANDS ARE PLEASURE MACHINES

And you thought it was all in the fingertips? Your palms, knuckles, nails, and even the webbing *between* your fingers all possess their own unique talents and texture. That means on any given night, you've got a full-on buffet of sensory selections to pick from. You could start with some stress-melting rippling on the shoulders, graze your nails down the back or chest, undulate your palm in "the wave" on the lower abdomen, throw in a playful slap or pinch on the posterior . . . need we go on? Our point is, use your hands well, and sex will never feel the same way twice.

HANDY FACT #2: USING YOUR HANDS DURING INTERCOURSE CAN TAKE SEX FROM COOL TO CRAZY IN NO TIME

While we think it's a no-brainer that better manual skills will come in handy during foreplay, what many people don't realize is that these techniques—even genital massage—can be done *during* intercourse, too. All it takes is a little reaching and/or clever positioning to be joined at the hip and have your mitts down there simultaneously.

And the effects can be incredibly climactic—especially for women, two-thirds of whom don't regularly reach orgasm through intercourse. The reason? A lack of stimulation to their main hot spot, the clitoris. We're not saying Big Os are the be-all and end-all of sexual ecstasy, but for those women who would like to reach peaks more often, lending a helping hand during intercourse can help improve the odds immensely.

HANDY FACT #3: GIVING YOURSELF A HAND DURING ORAL SEX CAN MAKE IT EXPLOSIVE

Oral sex can deliver some pretty sublime sensations, but as anyone who has ever licked his way to lockjaw knows, tongue muscles can tire. Meanwhile, fellatio fans face the problem that the average penis is five to six inches long, while the mouth is only two to three inches deep, past which the gag reflex usually kicks in. But just because we're saddled with these physiological shortcomings doesn't mean you just have to suck it up and suffer. Where the mouth and tongue fall short, your hands can easily pick up the slack. By mixing in a few manual moves between licks, you can allow your tongue to take breaks, or you can use your hands to cover more territory than your tongue could ever hope to reach on its own. During oral sex on a man, you can use your hand in conjunction with your mouth to create the illusion that you're taking him all in without it becoming a pain in the neck (literally). In fact, your hands are so adept at mimicking the sensations your mouth delivers that chances are, those on the receiving end won't even be able to tell where your mouth ends and your hands begin. And frankly, they won't care.

**HANDY FACT #4: USING YOUR HANDS ALLOWS YOU TO GIVE
YOURSELF THE OPTION OF SAYING "YES, TONIGHT DEAR"
EVEN WHEN YOU'RE BUSHED**

We have all had those days where we feel so overworked and exhausted that by the time we trudge to bed, it would take a crane to lift us into position for lovemaking. Maybe that's why one study by the National Opinion Research Center found that on average, one-third of Americans get it on only a few times a year, or not at all. But if, in theory, you would *like* to connect with the person lying catatonic next to you but just can't scrounge up the energy, consider hand jobs your low-impact, high-payoff alternative. No one has to climb on top and work up a sweat, or crouch below and head bob or tongue wiggle away. No, the only thing you'll need to move is your hands. Even just one of them is fine. With such an easy yet satisfying option at your disposal, those nights when you would usually roll over and say, "Not tonight, honey," might start looking up.

HOW THIS BOOK CAN MAKE YOUR SEX LIFE HOTTER THAN EVER

*If sex is such a natural phenomenon, how come there are so many
books on how to? —*BETTE MIDLER

Your hands are pretty nifty, but they don't run on autopilot. They need some guidance from that air traffic control center above—aka your brain. After all, your hands don't just *know* how to play the piano or type one hundred words per minute. These accomplishments are achieved with the help of teachers, how-to books, or instructional DVDs, and your skill will only start feeling "natural" if you practice, practice, practice.

While we largely accept this "practice makes perfect" proverb when it comes to work, hobbies, and other activities, we tend to brush this wisdom aside when it comes to sex. It's as if we just expect that the blueprints for getting it on are ingrained in our genes, in the same way that birds don't need to be taught to build nests or spiders how to weave webs. This may be true to a small extent. But we're talking *really* small—as in, maybe deep down humans naturally know to insert item A into slot B, or would at least figure it out in due time—but that's it. Any sex skill beyond that is learned, plain and simple.

HOW WE GOT SO HANDY WITH OUR HANDS

When strangers ask us, "So what do you do?" our answer often elicits raised eyebrows—and a ton more questions. The first is usually "What the hell is a sexological bodyworker?" First off, as you have probably guessed, we're not regular massage therapists. Such licensed professionals might know plenty about how to work out the kinks in your lower back, but they receive no training about how to handle certain choice areas below the belt. That's our area of expertise. But don't get the wrong idea here; we aren't running a seedy establishment where exotic women named Blossom or Bunny will give you a happy ending for a small fee. We don't *give* happy endings to our students; we teach people the hands-on skills they need to create their *own* grand finales, on a partner or on themselves (since operating your own equipment isn't always as easy as it looks).

Depending on the level and type of class we're teaching, students might be fully clothed, partially clothed, or au naturel—understandably an uncomfortable scenario for some, but those who brave their way through those first few awkward moments are often surprised how quickly they can relax and get to work. Some of the techniques we teach are as PG-rated as a shoulder massage; others are a lot racier. For example, did you know that rubbing the clitoris at two o'clock hits its most sensitive spot? Still other techniques may seem totally bizarre, but hey, don't knock a nostril massage until you've tried it. Our students leave armed with a newfound respect for their hands—by far the most underrated, underutilized instruments in their sexual arsenal (although not anymore).

And oh yeah—in case you haven't guessed, we're not *just* work colleagues. We're also a couple.

HOW THIS BOOK CAN COME IN HANDY

Ever since we met in a massage workshop in 2001, we have continued our "research," experimenting with new manual moves on each other (talk about a hard day's work). We also began teaching classes together, first just to a few friends, then to friends of friends, and the groups just grew from there. If it seems odd to you that people are hungering for instruction in something as simple as how to produce pleasure with their hands, we'd like to argue that it's *so* basic that people don't give it much thought at all, and thus aren't very good at it. Every day we see people botch even the simplest gestures of affection—witness awkward A-frame hugs, limp-lily handshakes—and in the bedroom, this discomfort is magnified tenfold. Perhaps that is why many of us shy away from learning even the basics of how to share the physical contact we all crave. We'd like to change that.

This book is for anyone—man or woman, singles or couples, gay, straight, bisexual, transsexual, or somewhere in between—who wants to improve his or her skills at the most elemental level at which we give and receive pleasure: touch. Here's what you can expect to learn in these pages:

- First, since in order to excel at the techniques we'll be teaching your hands will need to be strong, fast, flexible, and schooled in "palpation skills" (a snooty way of saying that they will be able to pick up the subtlest sensations), we have provided some exercises that will help make them fit for the task. And since great sex takes preparation, we have provided a checklist of things you should do to set the scene for a truly scorching encounter.
- Once your hands are ready to start causing trouble, we bet the first thing you'll want to do is reach for some pretty obvious areas south of the border. Not so fast. While it's easy to forget, the *entire* body is teaming with erogenous zones—ears, back, chest, butt, toes, nose, you name it—and a true master knows how to caress, massage, tickle, and turn on *all* of them. We'll give you plenty of ideas on how to do just that.
- Next, we'll teach you how to handle a man's ultimate hot spot— his genitals—in ways that will make him pinwheel-eyed with pleasure and plaster a grin on his face for days. The hand jobs he received back in high school won't hold a candle to what you're about to do to him.
- After that, we'll teach you how to caress a woman's nether regions with extraordinary results. This section may be especially eye-opening given that a woman's genitals are often trickier than a man's to figure out. In fact, many women come to our classes admitting they've never even had an orgasm, alone or with a part-

ner. Whatever the case, this book can help women experience their full pleasure potential.

- Finally, once you have these building blocks down pat, we'll show you some creative ways to incorporate your newfound handiwork into intercourse, oral sex, and more.

Let's face it: We could all stand to get a little closer to the people we love. And our hands may very well be the ticket.

1

GET YOUR HANDS IN SHAPE

I started out to be a sex fiend, but I couldn't pass the physical.

—ROBERT MITCHUM

First things first: Let's get your hands ready for all the excitement. Put a little effort into honing and toning their talents before you hit the sheets and you will be like a sports star who has taken care to train before stepping into the ring. If you want to be able to keep the pleasure going long into the night, then the solution is simple: Your hands need a little exercise.

Consider this chapter a personal training program for your hands. These miniworkouts (which are used by sexological bodyworkers and massage therapists) will make your hands stronger, faster, more flexible, and even more fine-tuned to feeling subtle sensations than ever before. What's more, they take only a few minutes to do and don't require a gym membership—any old place from your living room to your car is fine. For optimal fitness, each exercise should be performed at least once a day for one to two weeks to bring your musculature and sensitivity up to speed; after that, you can do them once per week to maintain your hands' pleasure-inducing performance levels.

While having to worry about getting yet one more body part into shape may seem like a drag, think of it this way: It's all for the pursuit of *pleasure*. What endeavor could be more worthwhile? Once you see the results, you'll be very glad you did these drills.

FOR STRENGTH

Exercise #1: Play Ball

Get a tennis ball, racquetball, or buy one of those squishy "stress balls" you often see strategically placed near the register at drugstores (no doubt to alleviate the mounting tension that comes from waiting for a prescription refill). Close your hand around your ball of choice and squeeze as hard as you can for three seconds, then relax. Repeat at least ten times. This will strengthen the muscles in your palm and fingers, helping you to knead your partner for a sustained session without wimping out.

Exercise #2: Towel Twister

This exercise will strengthen your wrists. Holding an end of a hand towel in each hand, twist the towel as much as you can, as if you were wringing water out of it. Hold for five seconds, then reverse directions. Repeat ten times.

Exercise #3: The Upper Body Booster

This exercise will increase overall upper body strength. Keeping your legs straight, bend over and place your palms on the floor so your body forms an upside-down V (if you have ever taken a yoga class, you may recognize this pose as the Downward Dog). Lean your weight onto your palms and press them into the floor, making sure to spread your fingers as wide as possible. Hold for ten seconds; repeat five times.

FOR FLEXIBILITY

Exercise #4: The Finger Stretcher

This exercise will stretch the muscles in each finger individually, as well as the corresponding tendons running down into the wrist. Holding one hand out in front of you, palm facing forward as if to say "stop" to oncoming traffic, grab its thumb with your other hand and pull it back for a second, then release. Then pull back your index finger, then your middle finger, and so on. Then switch hands.

Exercise #5: The Rubber Wrist

Pull your thumb down toward the inside of your wrist and hold for a count of ten. Then grab your four fingers and pull them back toward the top of your wrist for the same amount of time. Respectively this will stretch the top and bottom of your wrist for more all-around flexibility. Perform each stretch twice.

Exercise #6: The Forearm Flexor

Get down on all fours; the fingertips in both hands should naturally point forward. Rotate one of your wrists inward so your fingers are pointing back toward your feet. Then slowly lower your butt toward the floor; this will stretch the underside of the forearm you just rotated. Switch hands—and once you pull that off, try doing both hands together. Perform each stretch twice.

FOR DEXTERITY

Exercise #7: *Don't* Follow the Leader

Except for your thumb, whose raison d'être is to do its own thing (thus the term "opposable thumb"), the rest of your fingers prefer to stick together: If one moves, they all want to move with it. This follow-the-leader tendency can be a problem when you try to do certain techniques we teach that require a high level of dexterity, and that's where this exercise can help by forcing your fingers to break apart from the pack.

Here's how to do it: Gently rest your hand palm down on a tabletop. Lift your index finger one inch off the surface, then let it fall back to the table. Repeat ten times, then do the same thing with your middle, fourth, and fifth digits. Your ring finger, you'll find, is the weakest of the bunch. But over time all your fingers should improve.

Exercise #8: The Coin Flip

This exercise will also increase your dexterity, but be warned: It takes practice. That said, those who master this move will have a pretty cool party trick up their sleeve to impress random strangers. Extend your hand palm up, place a quarter on your index finger and then flip it onto your middle finger, then flip it onto your fourth finger, then your fifth, then send the coin back the way it came. Once you have mastered this move, try it on the knuckle side of your fingers instead.

FOR SENSITIVITY

Exercise #9: Hair Today, Gone Tomorrow

For this exercise you'll need a book, ideally one with really thin paper (a telephone book is ideal), and a long strand of hair. Open the book and place the hair on the center of any page; then carefully flip a page so it's covering the hair.

While you probably have a decent idea of where the hair is hiding underneath that page, pretend you don't—and force your finger to find it. Gently run your index finger across the page, feeling for the hair. Once you find it, flip a second page on top and see if you can still feel where the hair is. Continue adding pages until you can't feel the hair anymore. Then repeat the exercise with your middle finger, fourth finger, and pinky. The next time you try this exercise, push yourself to find the hair by adding even more pages. This technique will improve your "palpation skills"—aka the ability to pick up on very subtle sensations.

Exercise #10: The Balloon Press

This exercise will improve your ability to feel subtle differences in pressure, so that you can avoid pushing muscles in your partner's body past his or her comfort zone. Inflate a balloon, then slowly sink your fingertips into it. The surface should give pretty easily at first, less so as you press deeper. At some point you should feel the sensation shift from your *bending* the balloon's surface to *stretching* it. This change also occurs if you press your fingers into any muscle in the body (including those in the vagina and anus). At first the area will give easily, but if you keep going there will come a point at which you feel like you're stretching it—and since that can be painful, it's best if you don't cross that line. Practice on the balloon and you'll soon be able to pinpoint the difference.

Exercise #11: Armed and Ready

Once you have mastered the hair-in-the-phone-book and balloon workouts we think you're ready to try out one final exercise on the human body—either yours or your partner's. To start out, get your hand hovering a couple of inches over your (or your partner's) forearm, close enough so that you can feel the warmth emanating from the arm. Then, moving at a snail's pace, slowly close in so you can feel the arm hairs. Then close in further so you can feel the skin, then deeper until you feel the layer between skin and muscle, then even deeper until you can feel the muscle, then the bone. Then, just as slowly, loosen your grip and reverse your way back to your starting position, feeling for each layer as you go. Do this exercise slowly and it will hone your sensitivity in a whole new way.

2

SETTING THE SCENE FOR MIND-BLOWING SEX

Nothing can cure the soul but the senses, just as nothing can cure the senses but the soul. —OSCAR WILDE

As tempting as it is to reach straight for the genitals and start rubbing, let's not forget: Sex is a *full*-body experience. Focus exclusively on someone's privates and it's like playing a piccolo solo when you could be orchestrating a symphony's worth of sensations—one that permeates your sense of sight, sound, smell, taste, and touch in subtle, complex, and thrilling ways. To create an ensemble effect, a little preparation is in order.

Turning your typical bedroom into a well-equipped love den isn't as daunting as you might think. In fact, much of what you'll need may be in your home already, although you might not have thought to use it for *this* kind of occasion (you'll never look at your kitchen spoons the same way again). Some accoutrements we suggest you have on deck might seem obvious (like personal lubricant or massage oil), but the uninitiated tend to make grave mistakes picking which products to use, or where on the body to put them (and please believe us when we say you don't want to learn where *not* to put massage oil through trial and error).

To help ensure that you put together a bacchanalian buffet of sensory pleasures, this chapter is a checklist of things you should do or get before you start steaming things up. If you need to embark on a shopping spree, we have provided a list of Web sites in the Appendix, where you can find everything you need. Take these simple measures and your rapt audience of one will be tickled pink by all the sexy special effects.

WET YOUR WHISTLE: WHY WE ALL NEED LUBE IN OUR LOVE LIVES

If your hands are heading to your partner's privates, personal lubricant is a must. This slippery substance helps cut down on friction so your hands can glide over genitals in arousing ways—try making do without it and you may be in for a very rough ride. Using your own saliva might get you started, but unless you're a champion drooler, there's only so much spit to go around, plus it evaporates quickly. A woman's nether regions may lubricate naturally, but these resources can also run dry—even if she's turned on—due to medication she's taking, which stage of the menstrual cycle she's in, or even whether she drank eight glasses of water that day. Luckily, all of these problems are instantly solved with a store-bought stand-in. Just be sure not to use lube as an excuse to push past your partner's comfort zone; always check in to make sure he or she is enjoying what you're doing. There are three general types of lube to consider: water-based, silicone-based, and homeopathic. Here's a rundown of what they're like and which would be best suited for your purposes.

Water-based Lubes

True to their name, these lubes are made out of water, which means that they're safe to use with condoms and on women internally, unlike oils, which break down the latex in condoms and may cause vaginal infections. Water-based lubes are also inexpensive, won't stain your sheets, and come in a wide variety of flavors, colors, and textures. The one downside is they do tend to evaporate quickly, so you may have to apply more as you go or splash water on the area, which can reconstitute the lube you're already using. Still, overall, their popularity among sexually active sorts speaks for itself. Here are a few common brands:

K-Y Jelly: Many women have already been introduced to this lube at the gyno's office, where K-Y Jelly is used during pelvic exams to make them more comfortable. Since it's designed for doctors rather than lovers, K-Y tends to get sticky fast and is not our favorite. Still, there have been sexually enhancing improvements made on the original formula, and in spite of its downsides K-Y certainly has convenience going for it, as it's available in most drugstores.

Astroglide: So named because its inventor discovered it while working on the cooling system of the Space Shuttle, this lube tastes sweet and has a consistency similar to what the body produces naturally. The one downside: It contains glycerin, a type of sugar that can cause yeast infections in women who are prone to them.

Liquid Silk: It looks like moisturizer, it feels like moisturizer, and it lasts longer than any other water-based lube—a definite benefit if you feel that constantly reaching for another helping is interrupting your flow. It's also glycerin-free.

Slippery Stuff: In spite of its name this lube (which is also glycerin-free) is actually *less* slippery than most water-based brands. For those who prefer a thicker consistency, this one could float your boat.

Silicone-based Lubes
Long used on lubricated condoms, silicone is now sold by the bottle. Silicone lubes are more expensive than water-based varieties, but some argue that they're worth every penny. Since silicone doesn't evaporate, a little goes a long way—and can last for hours of fun. Eros and Venus are two popular brands, but just keep in mind that silicone lubes should not be used with silicone sex toys, since the liquid and solid forms will bind and ruin your toy.

Homeopathic Lubes
If you find that lubes tend to irritate your genitals or you're just extra conscientious about what's allowed on the premises, consider trying a 100 percent natural alternative. Sympathical, Sylk, and O'My are three brands we'd recommend. They're water-based and often contain extracts of fruits or herbs—and since they contain no artificial dyes, flavors, or preservatives, they're less likely to cause itchiness, irritation, or infections. They're also safe to use with condoms.

HOW TO KEEP SEX SAFE

We can't emphasize this enough: Protecting yourself against sexually trans-mitted diseases is paramount, especially if you and your partner aren't in a committed relationship or haven't been tested for STDs. While most people know they should use condoms during vaginal or anal intercourse and den-tal dams during oral sex, they're often unaware of what precautions they should take (if any) when it comes to using their hands. So here's the scoop. Generally, hand-to-genital contact is one of the safest ways to engage in sexual activities with someone. Provided there are no cuts or open sores on your hands, you're pretty well protected against HIV, chlamydia, gonorrhea, and many other STDs. That said, hand-to-genital contact does carry risks of transmitting herpes, human papillomavirus (HPV), which can lead to genital warts and other health problems. And if your hands have open cuts or sores, you are vulnerable to HIV as well. If you're concerned about any of the above, you can protect yourself and your partner by using latex, vinyl, or nitrile gloves. Just be sure that massage oil or any oil-based substance does not come in contact with latex, since oil will break down this material. To check for holes in gloves, inflate the glove by blowing into it then hold it closed and see if any air leaks out. If so, use a different pair.

*MMMMM*ASSAGE OIL: HOW IT CAN MAKE SEX MORE SENSUAL

Pouring massage oil onto your partner's body is similar to putting hot fudge on a sundae—it transforms an already good thing into a truly decadent indulgence. Massage is a great way to relax and warm up for phenomenal sex, and given that your hands should ideally glide over the skin rather than create so much friction they leave scorch marks in their path, it's best to keep a bottle of oil handy.

You can buy massage oil at spas, but be warned: You may cough up extra cash for the fancy packaging. So here's a little secret: You can buy the very same oils at a much cheaper price at your local health food store. Here are a few of the most popular types.

Coconut oil: Since coconut oil closely mimics the natural oils in your skin, it gets absorbed easily so you won't feel greasy, but it won't be absorbed so easily that you'll need to be constantly applying more. Plus it's antifungal, antibacterial, and has a long shelf life (many oils go rancid quickly). And let's not forget about the smell, which is bound to bring back fond memories of your last beach vacation and put you both in a pretty sexy state of mind. Coconut oil may also be used as a lube; it's our favorite. We recommend unrefined extra-virgin coconut oil for the best aroma and flavor.

Almond oil: Don't worry, it won't make you smell like a nut; refined almond oil is almost odorless. It also easily absorbs aromatherapy scents.

Sesame oil: This oil is often used in Ayurveda, the traditional medicine of India, and is reputed to improve circulation, constipation, bloating, and other health woes. It's thicker and can leave skin feeling greasy, but it can be blended with lighter massage oils to counter this tendency.

Grape seed oil: For those of you who would prefer a lighter oil, try this one, which is less greasy and is easily absorbed into the skin.

Avocado oil: This dark green oil is a little pricy, but it's worth it if you have dry skin and want to remedy it fast.

The oils we have just mentioned can be used on their own for a massage, but these so-called carrier oils can also be jazzed up if you mix in an essential oil. Extracted from certain plants, fruits, or flowers, essential oils are usually highly aromatic, which means a few drops will fill the room with a heady fragrance.

The benefits of using essential oils don't end there: A mere whiff of certain scents can have a dramatic impact on people's moods. So if you'd like to steer the evening in a certain direction, here's what to use:

To relax your partner: Cypress, lavender, orange, patchouli

If your partner is too *relaxed and needs a wakeup call:* Cedarwood, jasmine, peppermint (be careful with this one; use only a few drops)

To get your partner in a more amorous mood: Rose, sandalwood, vanilla, ylang ylang

Warning: Since essential oils are extremely concentrated, they should never be rubbed directly on the skin since they may burn like battery acid. Instead add a few drops to every ounce of carrier oil (or just read the directions on the bottle). And since essential oils evaporate quickly, make sure to cap the bottle afterward unless you want your first use to be your last. Some final pointers:

- If you're worried about the mess potential of massage oil and aren't in the mood for a big post-massage cleanup, there is an alternative: massage cream. It might not ooze sexiness like oil, but it won't spill and is easier to keep where you want it (on the skin versus on the sheets).
- Steer clear of household substitutes. Maybe you're wondering whether you can just grab the tanning oil/olive oil/moisturizer sitting around your home. But trust us: You'll regret it. For one,

olive oil and tanning oil aren't easily absorbed into the skin and will leave you feeling like you've been dipped in butter. Body moisturizers get absorbed *too* quickly; you'll mow through your entire jar of Nivea before the fun has even begun. Finally, in case you might want to kiss or lick any area you have touched, the chemicals and preservatives in tanning oil and moisturizer don't taste very good. All in all, unless you're truly desperate, save these items for cooking, tanning, and moisturizing.

- People with sensitive skin or allergies (especially to nuts) will want to carefully check the ingredients in massage oils and possibly avoid brands that contain dyes, perfumes, or preservatives. If you're not sure how you'll react to an oil, massage a tiny bit onto your wrist and leave it there for twenty-four hours to see if the area gets itchy or breaks out. If it does, that oil is probably not something you want to slather all over your body.

- We're not chemistry whizzes, but this much we know to be true: Massage oil and rubbers don't mix. That's because male condoms (and dental dams and diaphragms, for that matter) are usually made of latex, and latex breaks down in the presence of oil. So be careful to make sure that latex items stay well away from massage oils. Another option would be to use female condoms, which are made of vinyl and are safe for use with oil.

- Ideally, massage oil should not be used internally on a woman or on a man's genitals if intercourse might happen later, since the oil can linger in a woman's vaginal canal and possibly cause infections (the one exception to this is coconut oil, which is reported to keep the vaginal environment healthier due to its antifungal properties). Generally, your best bet for below-the-belt areas is a store-bought lubricant.

**LET'S GET COMFORTABLE: WHAT YOUR LOVE NEST NEEDS
TO STAGE SOME *VERY* HOT SEX**

Comfort is key to making a sensual experience sizzle, and not surprisingly, heading to bed is certainly a step in the right direction.
That said, a bed's surface may be too cushiony, and you might want a
little *less* give if you're planning to start off with a massage. If so,
throw down some blankets on the floor. A large futon on the floor is
another option; or if you become die-hard massage aficionados, consider buying a folding massage table. Granted, a good massage table
will run you at least a couple hundred bucks, but there are marked
benefits. Not only is there that nifty donut hole for your head (massage therapists call it a "face cradle"), the height is usually adjustable
so shorties and tallies alike can flex their manual moves at the ideal
elevation. And if you get to the point where you want to jump each
other, go ahead and climb on top. Collapsible or not, quality massage
tables are usually built to hold up to six hundred pounds and should
be able to handle some pretty rough use.

No matter where you decide to roll around, you'll want to make
sure to put down some bed sheets, especially if you're using massage
oil, since the stains are difficult to remove. If you're worried oil will
seep through the sheets, place towels or a waterproof picnic blanket
underneath. A second set of sheets can also come in handy for what
massage therapists call "draping": If your subject is shy about baring
all, throw a sheet over the body parts that need covering (you can also
cover areas of the body you aren't turning on so that they can keep
warm). When you throw these sheets in the laundry, keep in mind
that many detergents won't fully remove massage oil stains. Consider

using dish soap instead. Dawn, we've found, works especially well. To spot treat, place a dime-sized dab of Dawn on the stain and rub the material together before throwing it in with your regular laundry and detergent. Or add a teaspoon of Dawn per load along with detergent (do not use more, or you may end up with a bubbly disaster on your hands).

Last but not least, what your love nest needs are some towels of various sizes. Not only are they great for mopping up oil spills and other messes, but by folding and rolling them up in various ways you can create adjustable-size cushions to prop up body parts that'll appreciate the extra support. A rolled-up hand towel, for instance, can be placed under the neck; a larger towel can be wedged under a flexed knee. Comfortwise, some extra padding and support can make a huge difference and pave the way to a much more sumptuous experience.

YOU LIGHT UP MY LIFE: HOW TO GET YOUR GLOW ON

Lighting is crucial to a sexy ambience, which is why we think it's funny that most people restrict themselves to two choices: on and off. If you'd like to expand your options beyond pitch black or a harsh, I-can-see-every-pore-on-your-body glare, get a dimmer switch at your local hardware store. Don't worry, it's easy to install (instructions usually come with the dimmer, and the only tool you'll need is a screwdriver); it may be the best five bucks you'll ever invest in your sex life. With a dimmer switch you can adjust the lighting levels so they're low enough to set a mellow mood but bright enough so you can enjoy a little eye candy and read your partner's facial expressions, which is a surefire way to gauge whether your subject is happy, bored, or ecstatic over your efforts.

If you don't have a dimmer switch, turn on a table lamp and throw a light, colorful scarf over it (make sure it doesn't touch the bulb); this should work passably well in bathing the room in a warm, diffuse glow. Or break out some candles—flickering flames add instant atmosphere, so light one, a few, or a whole shrine's worth. We like to use candles made of soy or beeswax since your typical candles are made from petroleum-based paraffin, and the fumes can be unhealthy (ever seen how candles can blacken nearby surfaces? That gunk's getting in your lungs, too). Soy or beeswax candles, on the other hand, burn much more cleanly, which makes for better breathing. One final safety note: Don't fall asleep with the candles lit.

MUSIC TO MY EARS: TUNES THAT'LL TURN YOU ON

Nothing ruins an intimate moment like an untimely phone call from Mom, so make sure to turn off your phone, Blackberry, Treo, or anything else that might ring, beep, or interrupt the action. If you have an answering machine, turn down the volume (because long-winded messages from friends and family members can be equally libido killing). Unless you're a fireman, paramedic, or the president of the United States, whoever's trying to reach you can wait.

Now that we've nixed any potential distractions, consider popping in a CD or plugging in your iPod. Not only does music provide some mood-setting sounds; it may even alter the very *way* you two go at it. Beyoncé might inspire you to get the whole bed jiggling; jazz might get you improvising right along with those sax riffs.

CRANK UP THE HEAT: WHY YOU SHOULD TURN UP THE TEMPERATURE

It's all but impossible to melt into lovemaking if you're chilly, which is why we recommend keeping the room at a toasty 80–85 degrees (if turning up your thermostat isn't enough, use a space heater). Before you start rolling around, ask your partner if he or she is warm enough. Even if you're fine, keep in mind that everyone's ideal climate is different, plus the more active partner will generate more heat than the one who is lying still.

Also pay attention to the temperature of other things that could come in contact with your partner, namely, your hands (if they're cold, rub them together) and liquids like massage oil or lube. Rather than pouring oil or lube straight onto the body, consider heating it in the microwave, setting the container in a mug or bowl of hot water, or pouring it into the palm of your hand first to warm it up.

IS THAT A SPOON IN YOUR POCKET OR . . . ?
TOOLS THAT'LL TRIPLE THE FUN

Skin craves variety. In the same way your taste buds would rebel if you ate cheeseburgers for two weeks straight, the organ responsible for your sense of touch also prefers to feel a range of sensations. While your hands can provide an impressive medley of strokes and squeezes, why stop there? Consider using the following household items to caress, press, or tickle the skin and kick things up a notch:

Ice cubes
Feather
Spoon
Hairbrush

Silk

Satin

Velvet

Fake fur

Natural sponge

Loofah

Warm wet washcloth (kept in a bowl of steaming water)

CONDOMS: NEW USES FOR THE OLD RELIABLE RAINCOAT

Of course, you should keep condoms stashed in your nightstand if that's your method of birth control and to guard against sexually transmitted diseases. But what you might *not* know is that rubbers can be used in other ways. If you're up for exploring the back alley— aka anal penetration—putting a condom over your finger before you head in can help immensely on the hygiene front. For one, this will protect both partners from STDs. Two, since fingers that have been in the exit can't subsequently enter the vagina due to risk of infection, using a raincoat out back allows you to keep the fun rolling without a time-out to wash your hands.

While condoms may be the most widely available method to cover up before an anal excursion, there are alternatives, including dental dams (also known as latex shields), cleaning gloves (either latex, vinyl, or nitrile), and female condoms (which are made out of vinyl). Just remember, latex will break down if it comes in contact with massage oil, Vaseline, or any oil-based substance. If this limitation concerns you, stick with non-latex options. P.S.: We know female condoms haven't caught on like wildfire yet, but for what it's worth, we've tried them and give them two thumbs up.

3

A SENSUAL MASSAGE TO REMEMBER

"You look like you could use a massage . . ."

This single phrase has probably launched more sexual mayhem than all other come-ons combined. And for good reason: A thorough rubdown relaxes what's tense, perks up what's tired, and sends an unmistakable message to the brain that says, *Wow, that feels good. Give me more.* The perfect warm-up to more serious sexcapades, a massage can even convince people who swear they *aren't* in the mood to rethink matters a little. Even if your partner's bushed, stressed, or glued to a *Law & Order* marathon, try kneading his shoulders or rubbing her feet and watch the temperature rise.

Pretty much all massages feel good; your hands have a general idea what to do. Still, if you want to stand out from the sea of amateurs and give an extraordinary massage, this chapter will help you raise the bar. In addition to providing step-by-step instructions to giving a phenomenal massage, we have also addressed some key issues that people often wonder about but are too embarrassed to ask, such as *Does my recipient need to be completely naked? Should I strip down to my birthday suit, too? What if he pops a boner when I'm caressing his pecs? What if, out of the blue, she bursts into tears?* (Believe it or not, crying mid-massage is extremely common; we'll explain why it happens and what to do.)

STEP 1: SETTING SOME GROUND RULES

We know you're probably raring to strip down and get your hands wandering, but the very first thing you should do—and we know this sounds dull—is talk. Granted, giving a massage isn't like drawing up a UN peace treaty, but still, you'd be surprised how different people's expectations can be, and how awkward things can get if you find out mid-massage that you're not on the same page. For example, the massager for the evening might be thinking, *Boy, I'll bet the sex we're gonna have will be amazing!* Meanwhile, the massagee might be looking forward to getting a rubdown—period. Such misunderstandings will lead nowhere good, so that's why it's best to lay your cards on the table by broaching the following questions:

- What does your partner want to get out of the experience—to relax, get revved up for steamy sex, alleviate lower back pain, work out the kinks in a foot cramp, or something else? Massagers should also reveal their hopes and not despair if their dream scenario is light-years from their subject's. Try to strike a middle ground, or if none can be found the recipient should get his or her way and promise to return the favor later. Of course, once you've begun the massage and are in the thick of things, it's entirely possible one or both of you might change your mind.

That's fine (and we'll show you a tactful way to change course later), but still, it helps to air what you're thinking at the outset so you don't set yourself up for disappointment.

- Does your partner want to kick back and just enjoy the massage without lifting a finger, or would he or she prefer to take on a more active role and touch you, too? For that matter, do you even *want* to be touched? Some might actually prefer to focus 100 percent of their energy on giving without any distractions. While such a one-way exchange may feel a little strange since most sexual exchanges involve more give-and-take, consider trying it for a refreshing change of pace. You can have fun and even role-play—masseuse/client, maharaja/courtesan—if that allows you to more easily switch gears and embrace this new experience.

- What would you both like to wear—and bare? Clothing does tend to get in the way, so if you're both fine in the buff, great. However, if you're on the shy side, or have just started dating, or would otherwise like to maintain a little more mystery, then you might wear a bathing suit, pajamas, your stretchy yoga outfit, a sarong, or use what professional masseuses call "draping"—strategically placed bed sheets or towels that cover what needs covering but keep the body free from the constructing confines of clothing.

- How long will the massage last? Will there be breaks? Establishing a rough time frame is helpful for you since you can pace yourself accordingly and not get tired. But it's also beneficial for your partner who might get sleepy or, conversely, start feeling antsy. Knowing the time frame can help ease jitters.

- Would your partner like you to use massage oil or lubrication on the genitals? These are not the kinds of things you want to spring (or rather, squirt) on someone unawares. Also ask if your partner has any allergies or is prone to rashes or yeast/urinary tract infections so you can avoid products that might result in a nasty post-massage surprise.

- Are there certain areas on the body where your partner would like to receive a little extra attention? Even if as the massager you think the answer's obvious, ask anyway: You may be surprised to learn your guy loves having his ears rubbed, or that your gal's knees are her own personal sweet spot. Also ask if there are any areas that are best avoided. Some people are cursed with a ticklish stomach or feet so it would be pure torture to have these spots touched; others might just say that shoulder rubs just don't do much for them. Identifying these no-go zones clearly ahead of time not only will make for a more personalized, pleasurable massage, but will increase peace of mind, since the recipient won't have to worry that you may start heading in an undesirable direction.

STEP 2: SOME PRE-MASSAGE PREP WORK

Now that we've got all that yakking out of the way, you can start setting up shop. Here are a few other things you should take care to do before you dig in.

Trim/File Your Nails

Sure, long talons may have a certain sex kitten appeal, but they'll lose their allure pretty fast once they're gouging someone's shoulders. So do your partner a favor and make sure your claws don't extend more than a millimeter or two beyond your fingertips. If you're a nail biter, file off any scraggly, gnawed-off edges that might scrape the skin. If your hands are dry, massage oil (particularly coconut oil) will do wonders to soften them. To further sand down any rough patches, make a salt scrub by mixing one teaspoon of salt per one tablespoon of coconut oil and wash your hands with it.

Time It for When Your Partner Isn't Too Tired

Massages can turn even bright-eyed, bushy-tailed types into sleeping beauties. To avoid a snooze fest, schedule your session for a time when your partner will be awake enough to enjoy it.

Hold Off on Eating Until Afterwards

Heavy meals and massages don't mix well for a couple of reasons. For one, it's uncomfortable to have your stomach pressed if it's stuffed with a hoagie or half a pizza. Two, after you eat, your blood makes a beeline for the digestive organs, while a massage attempts to increase circulation *throughout* the body, which means you'll be fighting an upstream battle. So hold off on getting a massage for at least an hour after you've eaten, or at the very least, stick to light snacking, and plan a post-massage feast.

STEP 3: THE INS AND OUTS OF BREATHING

Breathing—you know, where you draw air in and out of your lungs—probably isn't something we need to remind you to do, during a massage or otherwise. Still, there are ways to enhance your massage experience through breathing:

Breathe Deep for a Better Massage

Many people breathe too shallowly while receiving a massage. Remind the recipient of the massage to take deep, slow breaths, inhaling through the mouth as if sucking on a straw and exhaling as if letting loose a long sigh. Many also make the mistake of inhaling just into the chest when the abdomen should also expand to fill the lungs to their full capacity. The deeper and slower the breathing, the more relaxed and pliable the body's muscles will be, and the more pleasurable the massage.

Breathe Together for a Deeper Bond

In some cultures, inhaling and exhaling in sync with someone is considered a bonding experience. In fact, according to the ancient traditions of the Maori tribe in New Zealand, it's actually considered *more* intimate than sexual intercourse. We're not sure if we'd go that far, but still, breathing together can be a way to get on the same wavelength and tune into each other's bodies on a whole new level. So try it for a few minutes at the beginning and end of your massage—with you following the pace of your partner—or for longer periods if you can. Or try a variation where one of you inhales as the other exhales. In Tantric traditions, a set of beliefs that aim to attain spiritual enlightenment through the body, alternating breaths is a way to exchange energy, maybe even merge souls a little. Don't knock it until you've tried it.

STEP 4: ASSUME THE POSITION

There's more than one way to give (and get) a massage, and since everyone's setup may be different—you may use a bed, the floor, or a massage table—it can help to know all your options. Here's the gamut, and while some are pretty obvious, there are tricks and tweaks to each that will make them considerably more comfortable for you both:

- Your partner lying on his/her front or back, with you strad-dling his/her butt or pelvis. If you're sitting around the thigh or knee area, make sure not to lean your full weight on those body parts.
- Your partner lying on his/her front or back on a massage table, bed, or other surface, with you standing to the side. For better leverage, keep a wide stance with your knees slightly bent.
- Your partner lying on his/her front or back, with you kneeling to the side. Since kneeling can be hard on your knees, put a pil-low under them or consider this non-kneeling alternative: Sit with one leg folded out as a prop and the other folded in. You can also sit in this position with your leg underneath your part-ner's head, which can feel very nurturing and be great for mas-saging the face, head, and arms.
- Your partner lying on his/her side, with you standing or kneel-ing on either side. This position is especially comfortable for pregnant women, who may find it uncomfortable or downright impossible to lie on their front or back.
- Your partner lying on his/her back, with you seated between his/her legs, which are bent and draped over your thighs. This position is great for people with lower back pain or tight ham-strings since it relieves tension in those areas. You can also raise your partner's legs so they're resting on your chest or shoulders.
- Your partner kneeling back on his/her haunches with torso and arms flopped forward onto the floor, with you standing and straddling his/her back. If you've ever taken Pilates or yoga, you might recognize your partner's position as the Child's Pose— and it does wonders for stretching and relaxing the back while you knead that area.

HEAVY PETTING: SOME GUIDING PRINCIPLES

In the next chapter we'll show you specific techniques to try on various parts of the body. But first let's fill you in on some general advice that will improve the overall experience.

Know How to Rub Someone the Right Way

An amazing massage boils down to a few basic strokes. Master these three and you're well on your way.

- The Glide. Using massage oil, press your palms and fingertips firmly into the recipient's flesh and slowly push away from yourself. Then circle back around to your starting point, either moving your hands back down the same way they came (as if you were painting a fence) or moving them in more of a long oval shape. The longer your stroke, the more soothing and relaxing it will feel for your partner; try it on his or her back, arms, chest, and legs.
- The Brush. Use your fingertips, fingernails, or the back of your hand to stroke the skin with the lightest, barely there touch. This technique tends to tease and turn on nerve endings, and can give your massage more of a sensual vibe. Try tracing circles on the stomach, breasts/chest, and face, or use this touch on the downstroke for The Glide. When you combine heavy strokes with feathery ones, the contrast will feel sublime.
- The Squeeze. Sore muscles will melt under this stroke, which works wonders on the shoulders, butt, and the back of the legs. Your hands should form a C shape for squeezing tissue in the space between your thumb and forefinger. You can alternate

kneading with one hand then the other, or squeeze your two Cs toward one another to knead even larger muscle groups (which is great for the butt). Just make sure to squeeze as much tissue as possible to avoid pinching the skin, since this can be painful.

Take It Slow

Moving a massage along at too brisk a clip is by far the most common error committed by amateurs. Try to match your pace to your partner's deep breathing pattern, only completing a squeeze or stroke every time he or she inhales or exhales (which can take anywhere from four to eight seconds depending on the state of relaxation). If your movements are making you breathe heavily or break a sweat, you're going too fast. Giving a massage shouldn't feel like a cardio workout. Also keep in mind that muscles take time to relax, so make sure you aren't pressing into them too quickly, which will only make them tense up. Instead allow your fingers to sink in slowly. Your massage should gradually build in intensity over time before tapering off gently at the end.

Don't Massage Too Hard—or Too Soft

Not surprisingly, men generally make the first mistake, squeezing women within an inch of their lives, while women's caresses are so gentle they barely make a dent in the knots in the neck. So be sure to check in with your partner to see how you're doing. Don't just ask, "How does that feel?" since most people will say "fine" or "good" out of politeness or because they might not know how good it *could* be. Instead ask, "Would you like it harder or softer?" That way your partner can voice a preference without feeling like he or she is critiquing your efforts.

Don't Freak Out if Your Partner Starts to Cry

Strange things can happen during a rubdown . . . like, suddenly, out of the blue, your partner starts dripping like a leaky faucet for no reason. Some massage therapists might theorize that you've stumbled across a spot on the body that has been storing painful memories and emotions; others might just say that a relaxing massage can bring down anyone's defenses. Either way, while your first reaction might be to think that giving this massage was a bad idea, on the contrary, crying is good. Think about it: People almost always feel better after a big bout of blubbering, right? That said, crying *can* be embarrassing—and it's your job to let your partner know you're cool with it. Only how?

Whatever you do, don't recoil in horror or ask, "What's wrong?" since this presumes there *is* something wrong and might make your partner feel even more uncomfortable. Instead look your partner in the eye, say, "It's okay" (which may bring on a fresh flood of tears), then ask, "Would you like me to continue or should we take a break?" If the time-out option is picked, try to maintain a little physical contact, whether it's holding hands or placing your palm reassuringly on one shoulder. This will subtly reinforce the idea that you're not weirded out by this impromptu sob-arama. In fact, going through it together might even bring you two closer.

Ease Out of the Massage Slowly

If all goes well, by the time you finish your massage (or whatever other shenanigans it may lead to), you'll have squeezed and kneaded your subject into a puddle of gratitude. At this point, the very last thing you should do is rush him or her back into the real world. After a massage, people can feel pretty disoriented; if they stand up too quickly they may feel wobbly or keel right over (believe us, we've

ON THE RECEIVING END? SOME THINGS TO REMEMBER

While the person giving the massage bears the brunt of responsibility for making sure the experience is a pleasurable one, the person receiving the massage also needs to know a few things.

YOU DON'T HAVE TO KEEP QUIET—Like sex, a massage is always better with a few sound effects. So go ahead and moan if you're so inspired, and if you have something you want to get off your chest, say it. A simple "That feels amazing" is always appreciated and helps steer your massager in the right direction. Or, if he or she is headed in the *wrong* direction, try pointing that out in a constructive way with "That technique you're trying on my shoulders doesn't do much for me, but I loved what you were doing on my lower back. Could we go back to something like that?"

YOU DON'T HAVE TO LIE STILL—Just because you're kicking back doesn't mean you have to act like you're paralyzed from the neck down. In fact, it can be darn sexy if you start to undulate your hips or reach up and start caressing your partner's face. If you're afraid your partner might be rattled if you start moving out of the blue, give a heads-up before the massage begins, or during the massage, say, "I feel like moving my hips a little, is that OK?" We'll bet you twenty bucks the answer will be "Please do!"

DON'T BE AFRAID TO SUGGEST A CHANGE IN PLANS—What can we say? People are wishy-washy, and that's okay. Even though you two agreed earlier that your massage would unfold a certain way, if you start getting other ideas while it's happening, go ahead and suggest a change in plans. Say, "I know we agreed that you would focus on me, but I just thought I'd let you know I wanna kiss you so much right now," or "I know I told you I'd rather not have sex, but this massage is so good it makes me want to throw you down on the bed and ravish you." Maybe your massager will be open to it, or, maybe you'll get back "Hold your horses, let's stick with the plan. We can do what *you* want later." But no matter what your massager's reaction is, it's worth getting your desires off your chest so they don't spiral through your mind in an endless feedback loop of *Should I say something? Would my partner be up for it?* Say your piece and see what happens.

RELAX AND ENJOY—It might seem odd that guilt may crop up during a massage, but it's fairly common to feel a little bad about kicking back while someone toils away pampering you like some modern-day sex slave. Or maybe you're uncomfortable being the center of so much attention, or worried that since your massager has focused 100 percent on you sans distractions, he or she is finally noticing your cellulite, or your hairy testicles, or how your nostrils flare when you're really enjoying yourself.

Oftentimes people will attempt to quell these feelings in a funny way: by reaching out and simultaneously touching their partner to even the playing field a little. If you suspect your motivations are along these lines, remember: (a) your massager is *not* noticing your cellulite, hairy testicles, flaring nostrils, or any other flaw you're obsessing about, (b) you'll have plenty of time *later* to return the favor by giving your partner a massage, and (c) your partner is probably enjoying the act of giving all on its own. Why provide a distraction? Instead allow yourself to indulge in the sensations your partner is creating without worrying about anyone but little old you.

seen it happen). So instead once you're done let your partner lie there for a while. Then your partner should sit up—but not stand—and swing his/her feet onto the floor for a few minutes. A glass of cool water can also help snap your subject back to reality. Recipients should stand up only once they feel ready.

4

A HEAD-TO-TOE GUIDE TO
ALL YOUR HOT SPOTS

MONICA: Now, everybody knows the basic erogenous zones. You
   got (starts labeling her diagram) one, two, three, four, five, six,
   and seven . . . okay, now, most guys will hit one, two, and three
   and then go to seven and set up camp.
CHANDLER: And that's bad?
RACHEL: Well, if you go to Disneyland, you don't spend the whole
   day on the Matterhorn.

—FRIENDS

Like rock stars, genitals get tons of attention. But let's take a moment to consider the rest of the body. As the gals on *Friends* so aptly point out, hot spots galore cover the expanse from head to toe. In fact, we'd say they undershot the mark, since by our count there are a whole lot more than seven erogenous zones worth visiting.

Given that your hands can flip each switch in a variety of ways, the turn-on possibilities are nearly infinite.

To get you started, this chapter contains more than fifty of our hottest techniques. Feel free to pick and choose which body parts and moves you want to try. Or, if you *really* want to impress your partner, follow this chapter step-by-step to treat your partner to the ultimate full-body massage. Done in its entirety, this rubdown is the perfect warm-up to more amazing antics. Try it and you may be surprised how many *ooohs, ahhhs,* and *omigod*'s ensue before you have even laid a hand on the genitals—or how explosive things will be once you do reach for the ultimate prize.

REV YOUR ENGINES: WHERE TO BEGIN

Ask your partner to lie facedown. Many of the body's large muscle groups lie along the backside—by relaxing them, you create the perfect foundation on which to build arousal later. While you can start your sensual massage at the head or the feet (feel free to ask your partner's preference), we're going to start at the head and work our way down. For most of these moves, you can either stand or kneel to your partner's side or straddle your partner's butt, a much sexier alternative. Remind your partner to breathe deeply before you get going. Here are some areas that are begging to be touched, and how to rub them right.

The Scalp

The scalp is rich in nerve endings, and it doesn't take a neurosurgeon to know that the more nerve endings there are, the greater the pleasure potential. To start firing things up, place your fingertips along

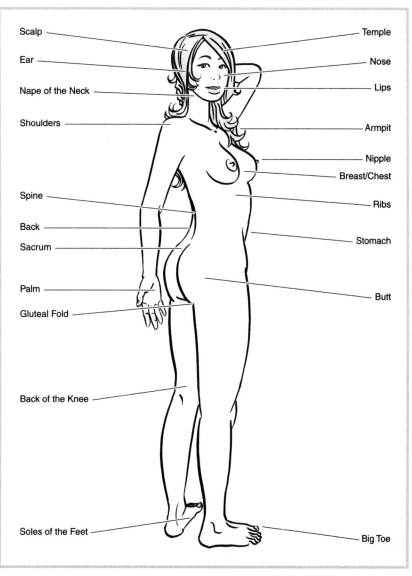

Scalp

Ear

Nape of the Neck

Shoulders

Spine

Back

Sacrum

Palm

Gluteal Fold

Back of the Knee

Soles of the Feet

Temple

Nose

Lips

Armpit

Nipple

Breast/Chest

Ribs

Stomach

Butt

Big Toe

THE BODY'S EROGENOUS ZONES

the hairline at the base of your partner's skull and start massaging the scalp in dime-sized circles as if you were washing your partner's hair. Slowly work your way up the scalp until you reach the front. For added measure, occasionally sift your fingers through your partner's mane like a comb, grip a chunk of hair near the roots, and gently tug (make sure you grasp enough hair that you're not pulling on just a few strands—that will hurt). Gently pulling on your partner's hair will stimulate the nerve endings *underneath* the skin's surface, where your typical scalp massage can't reach.

Nape of the Neck

This technique requires the steadiness of a surgeon, so for added stability, rest your right hand on your partner's right shoulder and your left hand on the left shoulder. Your thumbs, however, should remain free, and be perfectly situated to stroke the nape of the neck. Let your thumb pads move up and down along this extra-sensitive area like two sideways windshield wipers. Use a barely there touch that tickles the tiny hairs but not the skin underneath.

Once you have thoroughly tantalized the nape of the neck, inch your thumb up to the base of the skull and feel around for a tiny indentation. In Tantric traditions this spot goes by many names: the Bindu Point, the Mouth of God, and the Inner Smile since if you contract the muscles here (most easily done by wiggling your ears), this dimple morphs into a tiny U-shaped grin. Given that many muscles in the neck and skull are connected at this point, pressing down here with a thumb pad or massaging the area in tiny circles will relax the entire head and neck with almost zero effort on your part. Your recipient will want to breathe deep to enhance the effects and get in a deeper state of relaxation.

BONUS TIP TO TRY

This technique (which is done with your partner lying faceup) doesn't fit into our overall head-to-toe massage extravaganza, but it is a great one to try some other time. It's derived from cranial sacral therapy—a type of treatment used by chiropractors to balance cerebral spinal fluid levels, which can often get out of whack resulting in headaches, backaches, and other mood busters. Lucky for us, there's a spot on the back of the head that acts like a "reset" button that can reboot the body. To find it, make a fist with one hand and wrap your other hand around it. Then slide this mega-fist under your partner's head so the back of the skull is resting on it like a pillow. Hold that position for twenty seconds or until you notice your partner's breathing deepen, which is a sign that cranial sacral therapy is working its magic.

The Shoulders

Kneading the shoulders between thumb and fingers is nice, but the time is nigh to try a sexier, souped-up version. Place a hand on each shoulder and spread your fingers wide. Then press down in a rippling motion as if you were slowly playing the piano. This should produce a pleasurable tingling sensation while you work out the kinks. If you're doing this technique in our recommended position— you're perched on your partner's cute derrière—you can show how much *you're* enjoying yourself too by simultaneously circling your pelvis against the butt or tailbone. Consider it a steamy reminder of what's to come.

The Back

There are good back massages and then there are those that'll get your partner unwound and writhing in pleasure. To perform the lat-

---

BONUS TIP TO TRY

People who are tense tend to hunch their shoulders up to their ears. If you notice some evening that your partner fits that description, you can help crank him or her down a few notches by calling on your forearms for help. With your partner seated, place the bottom sides of your forearms on both of your partner's shoulders and press down, leaning your weight into them for a few seconds before you release.

To further relax the shoulders, stretch each one *while* you give them a rubdown. Gently tilt your partner's head to the left as you squeeze the right shoulder; have your partner take a few deep breaths to relax into the stretch before bringing the head back up. Then slowly tilt the head toward the right as you squeeze the left shoulder. Then slowly dip your partner's head forward toward his or her chest as you squeeze both shoulders at once.

---

ter, remain straddling your partner's butt (gyrating a little if you're so inspired) and place both palms on the base of the back above the butt. Firmly press the heels of your hands into the muscles alongside the spine and push up toward the shoulders. Once there, do U-turns outward and drag your hands back down (essentially your hands should be tracing two long, oval tracks on each side of the spine). Next move so you're kneeling at your partner's head and try this technique in the other direction, pushing your hands down the spine and back up. Unlike the previous position, this provides the additional benefit of stretching the lower back with each stroke.

Next move so you're standing or kneeling at your partner's side. The beefy back muscles can call for some pretty heavy pressure, so it's time to break out the big guns: your elbows. Place these pointy appendages on any fleshy area of the back and let them alternately sink in, *slowly*—this is key, since jabbing too quickly will cause the muscles to clench. Count to three as you gradually increase the weight, checking in with your partner about how much pressure is pleasurable. Then move on to another area that needs unknotting.

Place both hands underneath your partner's side at the bottom of the rib cage and pull up as if you were trying to lift the rib cage off the mattress or massage table. Then switch to the other side and repeat. This will not only knead the muscles running along the length of the rib cage, but can open the rib cage, allowing for deeper breathing and a greater state of relaxation. Add massage oil, and you can add a slide as you pull. And ladies, if your breasts "accidentally" brush against your partner's back during any of these maneuvers, all the better.

The Spine

Given that the spine houses the main cable of nerves that branch out into the entire body, it makes sense that stimulating this stretch would jump-start some sparks. Just make sure not to massage *on* the spine since that can be painful (generally, all bony protuberances should be treated with care). Here's how to hit the areas you want and avoid the ones you don't.

Straddling your partner's butt, create a U with your hand and situate it sideways at the base of the tailbone so your thumb is resting on one side and the edge of your pinky on the other. Then, pressing down firmly, push your U up the spine all the way to the neck, then release. The recipient should inhale as the hand moves toward the head and exhale as you remove your hand from the body. The sensation should create friction, with your thumb and pinky producing two parallel red streaks (watch your fingernails here; you don't want to scratch).

Next, with your palms facing down, cross your thumbs at the base so they form an X and your fingers spread wide like wings. With a light, barely there touch, run your thumbs up each side of the spine. Combined with the U above, this one-two punch of heavy then light strokes will get feel-good vibes blazing up the back. To steam things up even further, lean forward so your lips are inches from your partner's skin, then blow a soft, warm stream of air up the spine. Alternate with tiny kisses to get your partner squirming in anticipation.

The Sacrum

This triangular-shaped bone at the base of the spine contains the sacral nerve, which shoots straight into the genitals. So consider it your hotline to a good time (stimulating the sacrum can even give some men erections). Unlike other areas of the body, the sacrum actually enjoys some pretty heavy stimulation (just make sure to avoid the tailbone, which is located further down above the butt crack). To start heating things up, drum your fingertips on the sacrum. If that goes well, karate chop this spot with the edges of your hands. Finally, place your palm on the area, lean your full weight on it, and rock the sacrum back and forth (this is easiest if you stand or kneel at your partner's head). If you're unsure of how much pressure to use, go ahead and ask. We have generally found that people can't get enough and will say, "Bring it on, baby!"

The Butt

These two round mounds of flesh all but beg to be patted, pinched, and played with; now you're going to learn how to pay this area the homage it truly deserves. Standing or kneeling at your partner's side, place one hand on the top of one butt cheek and your other hand on the bottom. Then push your hands toward one another in a kneading motion, alternating hand after hand. After a few minutes, release and repeat on the other cheek. This technique accomplishes what one hand cannot: It kneads the *entire* gluteus maximus muscle, which is one of the thickest in the body and a major warehouse for stress retention. There's a lot of truth to the term "tight ass"—so it's good that you are loosening it up.

Our next point of interest is the gluteal fold, the crease at the bottom of each butt cheek. Using the pads of both thumbs, push into both creases until you feel a bony knob underneath. This is the sitz bone. Many of the muscles in your pelvis are attached at this point, so pushing down here for a few seconds can help relieve tension in the whole area and prime it for a good time.

Now that your partner's rump has been sufficiently tenderized, follow up with a light-as-a-feather caress. Still standing or kneeling to one side, lightly drag your fingertips across both butt cheeks, starting your stroke on the far side of the hips and ending on the side near you. Your hands should alternate and move in the same direction as if they were playing a harp; once you have "played" your partner one way, move to the other side and play it again.

Last but not least, straddle your partner's thighs and hold a butt cheek in each hand. Push them together for a few seconds, then gently spread them apart as far as your partner finds pleasurable. Next push one butt cheek up and the other down, then switch. This will stretch and stimulate not only the gluteal muscles, but an even more sensitive area in between them: the anus. Even if your partner has no interest in anything entering this exit, this technique will feel pleasurable. To show your partner you're enjoying yourself immensely as well, go ahead and grind your genitals against your partner's thigh;

men should also feel free to scoot up and press or rub their hard-on in the crease between their partner's butt cheeks.

The Legs

The first step to a good leg massage is to relax the hamstring, a large muscle on the back of the thigh. Straddling your partner's calf or calves, make a fist and place your knuckles just above the back of the knee. Using the weight of your upper body, roll your wrist forward so your knuckles ease into the flesh. Work your way slowly up one thigh.

Next wedge one hand under the knee and cup your palm over the kneecap. Then, with the fingertips of your other hand, trace a circle on the back of the knee—a well-known erogenous zone that requires only the lightest touch to be a turn-on. What's more, by touching both sides of this bony structure at once you allow sensations to sink through the area rather than just skim the surface.

After you have teased the knee, place your hands flat and parallel on each side of the calf and vigorously rub your hands back and forth, with one hand moving up while the other moves down as if you were trying to light a fire (if the leg in question is hairy, you may want to use massage oil so there isn't *too* much friction). Shimmy your hands up to the thighs to increase circulation and sensitivity from the ankles on up.

The very last thing you should do before moving to the other leg is to gently rock the leg you've been working on from side to side, starting with your hands on the ankle and slowly moving up to the hip. In the art of Tantsu, created by Harold Dull, rocking is an important way to lull your partner into a more relaxed and nurtured state. What's more, it may produce a slight rubbing sensation in the genital area that could also get your partner going.

THE FLIP SIDE: HOW TO TURN ON EVEN MORE TERRITORY

It's time to ask your partner to turn over so he or she is lying faceup. For some people many of the body's more heavy-duty erogenous zones are on the front side, so this is when you can start really steaming things up. Let's kick things off right by reaching for a Holy Grail of hot spots: the feet.

The Feet

A foot massage, as we all know, isn't *just* a foot massage. Perhaps John Travolta put it best while playing an overly chatty hit man in the film *Pulp Fiction:* "I've given a million ladies a million foot massages, and they all meant something. We pretend that they don't, but they do. That's what's so fucking cool about them." To make sure there's no mistaking *your* intentions (which are to get the sexual energy flowing, and good), let's start with the soles of the feet.

The soles of the feet are Reflexology Central—a metropolis of acupressure points that can get the whole body amped with electricity. To tap into these, place both thumbs on the bottom of one foot at the heel and paddle them into the flesh one after the other. Go slow (say, one thumb pad pressing into the flesh per second) and work your way up, making sure to cover every inch of the sole before switching to the other foot. Pay special attention to a spot between the big toe and second toe about two inches down. This acupressure point is called the Bubbling Spring, since pressing down here will cause energy to "bubble up" to the genitals and get things cooking in other ways.

Last but not least, let's not forget about the big toe—an appendage with special lust-inducing powers since according to Chinese medicine it is connected to the pituitary gland, an organ that is linked to hormone production. To activate, place a finger on each side of the big toe and roll it between your fingers. For extra kicks, lean down and suck on it (assuming it's nice and clean and the toenail is clipped, of course!). Women should also consider pressing their breasts against the soles of the feet and placing their nipples between their partner's first and second toes. If you like, ask your partner to pinch gently to give yourself and those toes something to write home about.

Once you have thoroughly amused your partner's little piggies, it's time to start slowly moving up the body. Consider repeating a few of the leg massage maneuvers you did while your partner was lying facedown. As you inch your way up, your partner may assume you're heading for the genital area. Tempting as that may be, try to resist the urge. After all, there are a slew of interesting destinations on the front of the body that we haven't even gotten to yet. So, if you can help it, bypass the genitals on the way up—a few strokes or licks are perfectly acceptable if you want to tease your partner a little—and head to our next point of interest: the face.

The Face

Caressing someone's face is Seduction 101: Not only will it win you major intimacy points; the sensation feels amazing. To start, place two fingertips from one hand on the right side of the forehead, and two fingertips from the other hand on the left side of the chin. Then lightly drag the fingers of both hands across the forehead and chin so that they're slowly traveling in opposite directions. Once your fingertips reach the other side, head on back. Since your hands are traveling in opposing directions, the sensory receptors in the face will perk up and become intently tuned in to every move you make. Next try the same technique but with the back of your hands. The rougher texture will make the same move feel entirely different—and the contrast will help keep those nerve endings titillated.

The Eyes

The skin around your peepers is so delicate you'll want to use the lightest caress here. For this purpose you're best off using the fourth finger, since it's weaker than your index or middle digit and therefore ideal for doling out feathery strokes. Ask your partner to close his or her eyes, and then place your fourth fingers on the inner corners of the eye sockets. Very lightly drag your fingers out along the lower lids, around the upper ones, and back to the starting point. Do this ten times then repeat in the other direction.

The Temples

Let your massage flow from the eyes to the temples—an area that typically holds a lot of tension. While massaging this area with your fingertips can help ease someone's angst, you can also zap stress here in a more surprising way: by pressing your fingertips on both sides and gently jiggling your hands back and forth, moving the skin with your fingertips but keeping your actions minimal enough that the head remains stationary. Unlike your usual stroking motion, this technique sends reverberations into the skull, resulting in a deeper state of relaxation.

The Ear

As far as erogenous zones go, the ear is a classic. According to Chinese medicine, the ears contain over 120 acupressure points that are connected to all areas of the body. That means that by firing up the ears, you're essentially stoking the coals everywhere at once. To kick-start this sexy chain reaction, use the tip of your index finger to lightly trace the outer ridge of the ear from the top where it meets the skull on down. Once you reach the earlobe, take it between thumb and forefinger and gently massage the area in tiny circles. Given that the center of the earlobe is linked to the heart, this massage could subtly stir up some lovey-dovey feelings.

Next hold the earlobe between thumb and forefinger and gently pull, then slowly swing it back and forth like a pendulum. This isn't so much for your earlobe's enjoyment as it is to stretch and stimulate the nerves *inside* the ear canal that your fingers can't reach (nor should they try, either). This virgin territory is an untapped cavern of sensitivity.

The Nose

Most people generally don't think of their schnoz as an erotic area, but it *is* an orifice (which is inherently erogenous), has the second highest number of nerve endings on the face (next to the mouth), and last but not least shares one striking similarity with your genitals: erectile tissue. Don't worry, the effects occur *inside* the nasal passages, so no, turning it on won't make your partner look like Bozo the Clown. All we're saying is that your sniffer is designed to respond to a whole lot more than a whiff of perfume or a pot roast.

So how exactly do you stimulate the nose? Bear with us, since this is going to sound weird: While jamming your finger up someone's nostril might sound more like a toddler's prank than a turn-on, it's worth a shot. According to Taoist traditions, the body is full of "energy circuits" that cycle *chi,* or life force, through the body. One such circuit passes right through the nostrils, and by gently inserting one finger

BONUS TIP TO TRY

If your partner has a headache or earache, pinch the tragus—the nub of cartilage in front of the ear hole—and pull laterally. According to Chinese medicine, this will alleviate most noggin-related ailments, which means you have the perfect solution to that old "not tonight I have a headache" excuse.

and squeezing the outside of the nose between thumb and finger, you can tap into this loop and feed off each other's energy. If you're feeling especially adventurous, try this with your tongue instead of your finger. You can jack into this same energy circuit one story down by touching the roof of the mouth about an inch back from the teeth.

The Lips

Using just the tip of your index finger, trace a trail around the outer edge of your partner's pout. It may not seem like much, but less is often more when you're trying to titillate this extra-sensitive area. For extra passion points, linger around the philtrum, that cute little indentation above the upper lip. The ancient Greeks deemed this spot the most erogenous zone on the body, and modern science seems to support this claim. Two major cranial nerves lie close to the surface here, making this tiny area a hothouse of sensitivity.

Cute as that kisser is, though, it doesn't always need to be treated with kid gloves. To up the intensity, pinch your partner's bottom lip between thumb and forefinger and roll it between your fingers. Sure, it may seem cheeky (and probably isn't something you'd want to try on a first date), but doing so brings blood flow to the area and gets those nerve endings buzzing anew.

BONUS TIP TO TRY

Since it's hard to feel sexy when you've got the sniffles, here's what to do if your partner's stuffed up. Place your index fingers on each side of the bridge of the nose between the eyes. Massage three tiny circles here. Then do the same on the divots on each side of the nose above the nostrils. Stimulating these four pressure points can help relieve sinus-related woes.

Finally, insert your index finger into your partner's mouth and run the tip along the teeth and gums. Twist your finger around their tongue, playing a game of cat and mouse. Voilà, you're French-kissing with your finger. You can top off all this lip teasing with a long, deep mouth-to-mouth kiss to whet your partner's appetite for more.

The Chest

The chest is an erogenous zone extraordinaire. You don't even have to touch it to turn it on. Just hover your hand about a millimeter above the skin and let it drift over these peaks and valleys. It's okay if you sometimes lightly brush the skin, but even without direct contact your partner will *definitely* feel it.

Once you have titillated those nerve endings, it's time to stretch the area. Cup a breast or pec in each hand (hold the nipple between index and middle finger for added maneuverability) and squeeze the breasts or pecs together for three seconds, then spread them apart, then move them in circles. While you have probably never considered stretching the chest/breasts, it's an incredibly relaxing sensation that can expand your partner's pleasure potential.

Now that you have turned that bosom to butter, pour massage oil on the area and treat it to a massage. Place your hands between the breasts and stroke down, around, then up the sides in circles. Not only will this massage feel amazing, but it will improve the flow of blood and lymphatic fluid to the area. And over time it can lead to even more eye-popping results: According to Taoist beliefs, massaging the breasts in this manner will make them grow in size. We're not talking Dolly Parton proportions overnight, but if you keep at it (Taoists say 108 rotations per day is optimal), you can increase that bust by up to two inches. This technique is equally effective on men or women, although women may find the size-altering effects of particular interest. If, on the other hand, your goal is to shrink that bosom down a bit, perform the massage described above in the opposite direction. This will stem the flow of blood and lymphatic fluid to the area, and while it won't turn melons into apples, it may make a difference—and feel really good to boot.

You can caress, stretch, and massage the breasts in just about any position, but we highly recommend that you do these moves straddling your partner's pelvis. Why the heck not? Just because you're holding off on lavishing attention on the genitals until the very end doesn't mean you can't have a little fun rubbing against each other while you wait.

The Nipples

The chest may be fun, but the nipples are party central. To turn on those high beams, spread your five fingers out on each breast as if they were the spokes on a wagon wheel with the nipple at its center. Then slowly draw your fingers in toward the nipples and release *just* before you hit nipple territory. Even though you're not stimulating the nipples directly, the sense of anticipation alone will get these two hot spots humming.

Next lightly stroke the nipples with your fingernails. Once your talons have gotten their attention, switch to rubbing the nipples with the palms of your hands. The stark contrast between these two sensations will heighten the impact of each, making those scratches seem even more devilish, those palm strokes more soothing. Finally, try pinching the nipples, then slowly pulling them away from the body as far as your partner likes it. Ask your partner to inhale and exhale deeply while you hold the stretch. In doing so you increase blood flow to the area, resulting in stronger, harder nipple erections.

The Armpits

They sweat and often smell, and yet buried in their depths lies a reason to brave the trip: polarity points—nerves that, according to Chinese medicine, are associated with certain types of energy that travel up to the brain and affect your outlook. Press on these spots (just ask your partner to lift an arm then press your thumb in dead center for ten seconds), and you can "block" that energy and change someone's attitude toward many things—including how he or she treats *you* in bed. Which pit to hit depends on your partner's current mental state. For people who are stressed and "in their head," press on the right pit. This will block the passage of "masculine" energy, the result being a more sensual, emotional lover. If, on the other hand, your partner tends to be too shy or overly sensitive, press on the left pit. This will block the passage of "feminine" energy, and turn timid sorts into tigers.

The Arms

These limbs are like the wallflowers at a high school dance: They rarely get much attention, and yet if you give them a chance, you'll find it doesn't take much to get them smoldering. To rouse them, stand or kneel at your partner's side, then take his or her hand nearest you and tuck it under your armpit. That way, it can stay raised but relaxed at the same time. Then, using lots of massage oil, wrap both of your hands around the forearm and slowly slide your way up. Once you reach the shoulder, circle back down. Next do the same stroke only switch to using just your fingernails. In particular, the extra-sensitive inner arm will find the feel of your nails a turn-on.

The Hand

Take your partner's hand in yours and, using the index finger of your other hand, lightly trace circles on the palm. Then go a little deeper by pressing your thumb into the palm and massaging in dime-size circles, moving the skin with your hand so you're kneading the muscles underneath. The palm is packed with not only nerve endings, but acupressure points that can send pleasure rushing to other parts of the body.

Next up: the fingers. Interlace your digits with your partner's so the webbing between your fingers is snuggled up against theirs. Then, squeezing tightly, slowly inch your hand upward and off the fingertips. By doing so you'll increase blood flow to the fingertips and make them tingle (try this with massage oil and it will feel especially sensual). Last but not least, the outer edge of the pinky is a point of special interest, since it is considered a tertiary erogenous zone that feels pleasure once someone is already aroused. So if you have already kindled some heat (which will definitely be the case if you've been following this chapter step by step), head to the pinky to add fuel to the fire. Use the edge of *your* pinky to rub the side of your partner's in a soft, light sawing motion.

The Stomach

Whether it's a six-pack or a little soft around the edges, the stomach is a sexy, and sensitive, area of the body that will appreciate what you're about to do next. Using the flat of your palm, rub wide circles around the navel in a clockwise direction (up your partner's right side and down on the left). This is the same direction food travels in the intestines, so in essence you're helping move things along, which can help alleviate cramps, constipation, gas—and, in the process, clear this person's dance card for more erotic endeavors.

One spot on the belly worth a second visit is the Sea of Tranquility—a set of three reflexology points a few inches below the navel, so named because this area is considered the epicenter of your sexual and creative energy. Lightly caress it with your fingertips or place the flat of your palm just below the navel and undulate your hand in a wavelike motion. This will boost blood flow to below-the-belt areas—and a good thing, too, since that's where you'll most likely be heading next.

Now that you have induced a state of relaxation and revved the arousal levels, your partner will probably be very, very ready for you to take things further. The next four chapters will help you do just that, showing you how to put your hands on that pièce de résistance in your partner's pants with mind-blowing results.

5

HOW TO GIVE HIM A HAND

God gave man a penis and a brain, and only enough blood to run one at a time. —ROBIN WILLIAMS

Nothing—and we do mean nothing—turns a man's mind to mush like a few strokes on his genitals. In fact, many of you may find it so easy to make men speechless with lust that (admit it) you take your powers for granted and have gotten a little lazy. Like straight-A students who never study, you coast through your sexual experiences never really learning in detail what makes his twig and berries truly tick. After all, if what you're doing already puts a smile on his face, what more is there to know?

We won't argue with the fact that a man's genitals are amazingly user-friendly. Still, guys *do* know the difference between good sex, great sex, and an *oh-my-God-I'm-in-heaven* erotic encounter, and the only way to pull off that third steamy scenario is to ditch your usual mattress moves and broaden your horizons a bit. There are countless ways to "spice things up" in bed—dirty talk, chocolate sauce, or greeting your honey at the door dressed in Saran Wrap, to name a few. Sure, men may find these prospects titillating. But let's face it: Far more essential to a satisfying sexual experience is how well you're stimulating his privates. This is one area where your hands excel. Combine their deftness with a little knowledge of his anatomy below the belt, and you're armed and ready for one helluva hot night.

On that note, let's take a good, long look at his goods. The more familiar you are with his hardware and how it works, the easier it will be to perform all sorts of sophisticated techniques to turn it on, keep it on, prevent it from exploding too soon, and more.

AN EYE-OPENING MAN-ATOMY LESSON

In spite of its apparent simplicity (and the questionable nicknames attributed to it), a man's Mini Me is much more complex than most people have probably ever considered. For instance, while the full monty is usually seen as one giant homogenous hot spot, the reality is that certain points are sensitive, others less so, and still others are so touchy that only the lightest finger wiggle will set them loose. Here's a rundown of the areas you'll encounter, as well as the best way to handle them.

The Shaft

We think it's pretty self-explanatory what part of the penis we're talking about here, and it's probably the first thing you grab once

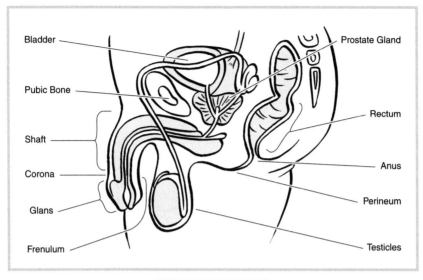

Bladder

Prostate Gland

Pubic Bone

Rectum

Shaft

Anus

Corona

Perineum

Glans

Frenulum

Testicles

THE MALE GENITALS

you've peeled off his skivvies. That said, for all the time you spend with your hands wrapped around this pillar to pleasure, it's actually one of the *least* sensitive areas of his anatomy. That doesn't mean you should steer clear, merely that you're better off concentrating on bolder strokes. In fact, go ahead and gently slap, stretch, and squeeze it to see how he likes it. Once you feel like breaking out some subtler handiwork, inch your grip up to our next point of interest.

The Glans

Usually referred to as the head of the penis, this acorn-shaped area is like the penthouse suite as far as fun is concerned. Since it contains hundreds more nerve endings than the shaft, it's highly sensitive—

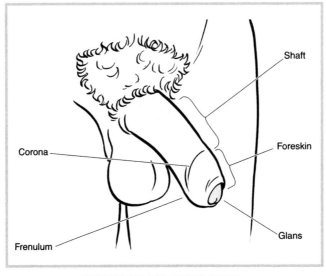

THE UNCIRCUMCISED PENIS

even the lightest caress can send shivers down his spine. You should take care not to polish this apple *too* vigorously, since it can easily become overstimulated, resulting in numbness or pain rather than pleasure.

The Corona

This is the ridge where the glans meets the shaft. Many of the nerve endings in the glans are concentrated along this loop, so it's totally worth lingering on this lip. Certain points on its circumference may be especially sensitive; to find out where, treat the corona like a clock face and make the rounds, rubbing every hour, on the hour. You may find six o'clock of particular interest (more on that next).

The Frenulum

If the penis has a sweet spot, this is it. Located on the underside of the corona, this point is a powder keg of pleasure that can be ignited with a mere pinky wiggle. In our classes, we have found that only half of our male students have a clue that this extra-sensitive area exists— and only a handful of them know it's called the frenulum. If your partner's in the dark, how grateful do you think he'll be if you make the introduction?

The Foreskin (If He's Uncircumcised)

Men who aren't circumcised naturally have more for your hands to please: the foreskin, an extra layer of tissue that covers the glans like a skullcap. Encountering one for the first time can be a little baffling, but this perplexing carapace comes with some unique arousal-inducing benefits. For one, the skin here is rich in a special type of nerve receptor called Meissner's corpuscles whose sole purpose is to feel pleasure, period. Secondly, by moving the foreskin up and down, you can stimulate both the glans and its covering, doubling his pleasure. Once the penis becomes erect, the foreskin will retract, at which point you may be able to treat the penis similarly to circumcised models. Still, to be on the safe side, ask your partner for a little direction.

The Testicles

Given that future generations of the human race depend on these two little sperm factories, it's understandable that a man's family jewels should be handled with care. Yet many people make the mistake of avoiding toying with the twins entirely, which is a shame since his cojones contain tons of nerve endings that are starved for some attention. Many men will enjoy it if you lightly caress the testicles with your fingertips, cup them in your palm and jiggle, or even pinch and pull on the scrotum—the pouch of skin that encases this valuable merchandise. The only two things you *should never* do is twist (which will pinch the vas deferens, the tube through which sperm travels into the penis) or squeeze. A good rule of thumb is to treat the testicles like eggs you don't want to break. So start gently, check in with him for feedback, and if at some point you feel his testicles contract and rise toward his body, congratulations! That means he's enjoying what you're doing. Take note and continue.

The Perineum

This area between the testicles and the anus, also quaintly known as the "taint" since " 'tain't one or the other," is a largely untapped erogenous zone that you should start cashing in on pronto. Buried beneath this spot is the prostate, a supersensitive gland. You can jump-start all kinds of hijinks when you press on the perineum and turn on the prostate. The prostate can also be stimulated via a more direct means that we'll discuss next.

The Anus

The anus is often treated like the bad kid on the block that shouldn't be played with, but those who hazard this side of the tracks will find its bad rap is largely unmerited. Next to his johnson, this area is decked out with more nerve endings than any other area of the body. And if that weren't enough of a reason to explore, about three inches inside this aperture you'll encounter a walnut-shaped bump—the prostate gland, a wellspring of sensitivity that can set off even more sparks.

HANDLING HIS ULTIMATE HOT SPOT:
SOME GUIDELINES TO KEEP IN MIND

In the next chapter we'll discuss specific techniques to try on the above-mentioned man parts that will blow his hair back and leave him begging for more. But before we get to that we feel it's best to start off with some overall pointers. Giving great hand is not as simple and self-evident as it is often made out to be. Heed this advice, and you'll avoid a few common misjudgments and leave his peter very impressed.

Don't Expect a Raging Hard-on the Whole Time

Boners are funny that way: Sometimes they pop up with no encouragement whatsoever (and when they're least convenient to deal with); other times every trick in this book won't inspire an inch of interest. Either way, don't assume you're wasting your time if the tent pitching is taking a while, or if his Maypole rises but then starts losing altitude. While people are conditioned to think that erection = arousal and use it as a barometer of their success in the sack, as any guy will tell you, the penis truly has a mind of its own. So don't take its actions (or lack thereof) too personally.

Meanwhile, remember that firm or flaccid, his love rod still contains the same number of nerve endings that can register on his Richter scale; some men (especially older gents) can even ejaculate when they're soft as a sundae. In fact, many of the genital massage techniques we teach are best performed when his hard-on is anything but. No matter what, if you find yourself face-to-face with one that refuses to roar to life, probably the worst thing you can do is stop and ask, "Is something wrong?" Penises don't respond well to pressure, so your question will only feed your partner's mounting performance anxiety and keep liftoff in limbo. Instead ask, "Does this feel good, or would you rather I try something different?" Your partner may steer you in a better direction, or reassure you that while things might not look like it, he's having a grand old time. Either way, eventually things should start looking up.

Request a Hands-on Demo

If you have never watched your guy masturbate, now is the time to ask (or, if you have already, appeal for a repeat performance). Every johnson is a little different, and the only person who knows a certain model's particular quirks is the guy behind the wheel. To get the inside scoop, you could of course ask him to pontificate about his likes and dislikes. But actions speak louder than words, so ask him to *show* you how it's done and you'll get a real eye-opener.

Understandably, some men might be bashful about performing this typically private act in front of you. If he's reluctant, suggest a two-way performance where you both masturbate in front of each other; few red-blooded men would be able to resist such an offer. Another alternative is to put your hands on his privates, layer his hands on top of yours, and have him guide you through the movements. However you conduct your tutorial, you'll learn tons about where and how he likes to be touched that you can file away in your memory bank for future use.

That said, don't copy his actions completely. In case you didn't know this, most men (even those in relationships) masturbate far more than you'd care or dare to imagine, and for all kinds of reasons—because they're horny, because they're bored, because there's a commercial break during the NBA playoffs—all in all, just about any occasion can be seen as an opportunity to jack off. As a result, many men don't raise the bar very high when tugging their wares—and it's up to you to show him how good it can get. So if you do get to watch him masturbate and are a little surprised to see his hand pumping at breakneck speed, that doesn't mean you should follow his lead to a tee. Consider his actions a general framework, within which it's your right and duty to add your own personal touch.

The Penis Can Withstand Some Pretty Rough Play

Ever seen Penis Puppetry? It's a performance where guys get up on stage, whip out their "puppets," and start bending, squashing, and all but tying them in knots to form hamburgers, Windsurfers, or whatever else they can imagine fashioning for their own and others' amusement. Our point isn't that you should book tickets to the show (although you should because it's quality entertainment), but to prove to you beyond a doubt that a man's genitals are sensitive but by no means delicate. That's right, his genitals can be folded like origami, flattened like pancakes, and stretched like Silly Putty, no problem (well, maybe that's pushing it a bit, but you get our point).

While a man's genitals are especially pliable while in repose, hard-ons can also be gently bent (at the base) without adverse effects. Even the testicles aren't as fragile as most people think. So if you're treating his genitals with *too* much loving care and concern, you could be shortchanging your partner out of a range of lovely sensations. So don't be afraid to push that penis around, test the boundaries, and see what *he* tells you is too much, rather than trying to second-guess where his pain threshold lies. As long as you proceed slowly and check in with him, you'll be amazed where your creativity may take you, and how much he'll enjoy it.

Balance Pace with Pressure

Sure, men may act like they could never get enough of you rubbing right where it counts. Still, *too* much stimulation will numb his nerve endings. To avoid going overboard, respect the yin and yang relationship between pace and pressure: The tighter your grip, the slower you should go; the looser your grasp, the faster your fingers should fly. And if you have been tending to the highly trafficked head and shaft for a while, give it some downtime to recharge and move on to another area of his anatomy. Play with his balls, stroke his pecs, or even (here's a novel idea) head all the way up and give him a long, lusty kiss. Men dig the romantic, mushy stuff much more than they'll ever let on.

Sex and Drugs Don't Mix

Whether he's had a few beers, a bong hit, or something stronger as a prelude to your evening à deux, just know that while most of these substances may loosen inhibitions, they can also slow circulation (which is why, as you have probably noticed, men have a hard time getting it up when they're drunk). Smoking also stems blood flow, and even prescription medications—most notably antidepressants—can throw a wrench in his ability to get it up, keep it up, or move it on out. If he suspects his meds are slowing him down, he can talk to his doctor about switching to a drug with fewer sexual side effects.

Experiment with Different Positions

There's more than one way to situate yourselves during the hands-on action, and each has its charms. Here are some ideas on how to get comfortable:

- He lies on his back with his legs together while you straddle his thighs. He can also spread his legs and have you kneel between them, which allows for better access to his testicles and anus.
- He lies on his back with his legs raised and the backs of his knees or his feet on your shoulders while you sit on the mattress below his butt with your legs spread in a V to each side of his body. Since his rear end is elevated, this offers even better access to his nuts and bolts out back.
- He sits and you are seated next to him or kneeling between his legs—an especially adoring pose from his vantage point since it makes him feel like a king.
- He stands and you sit or kneel in front of him. Since this position forces him to tense his thighs and buttocks, this can add *oomph* to every sensation. His legs can be together or spread apart.

Make Sure He's Not Holding His Breath

As the action heats up, many men tend to tense their bodies and hold their breath—a common impulse if they're trying to concentrate. But the fact is, muscles and nerves need oxygen to function properly. The more he breathes, the more he can feel, so remind him to inhale and exhale deeply to keep the hot-blooded fun flowing.

Take Your Sweet Time

Admit it: It's pretty easy to get a guy to reach Kingdom Come, whether that's via your hand, mouth, vagina, armpit, or otherwise. And sure, when you're tired or time is tight it's tempting to move things right along because you can (and you won't hear him complaining). We're not saying these quickie climaxes aren't nice. But given that the strength of his sexual release is directly correlated to how wound up you get him beforehand, why settle for a molehill when you could shoot for Mount Everest peaks? To build his pleasure, try slowing down the pace of your heavy petting. Or if he's close to the edge, keep him teetering on the brink with a little teasing. It's definitely time well spent.

Is He About to Blow? Tips to Prolong the Fun

You're probably familiar with the Point of No Return—that moment when a guy is mere milliseconds away from experiencing a small piece of heaven on earth. While its very name suggests there's no going back at this juncture, it actually *is* possible to slow him down if you want to draw things out. If he makes it clear in so many words or groans that he's near Nirvana, wrap your thumb and forefinger in a ring around the base of his testicles and gently pull them away from his body. The reason this works is that prior to ejaculation, his balls hunch closer to the body to prepare for blastoff. By pulling them away from their locked-and-loaded position, you can keep his barrage at bay almost indefinitely. Don't worry, it won't hurt; it merely delays the big launch until you both decide the time is right.

Yes! Yes! Yes! How to Make Your Man Multiorgasmic

You're probably aware that women can experience multiple orgasms, but here's a newsflash you might have missed: Men can be multiorgasmic, too. With a little training, guys can hit two, three, or more

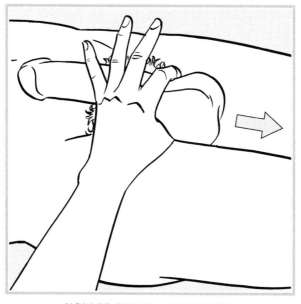

HOW TO DELAY EJACULATION

high notes without taking long time-outs in between. If you're dubious, allow us to explain the science behind this bold claim.

It's often thought that in men orgasm (the pleasurable contraction of muscles) and ejaculation (the release of semen) are all wrapped up in one big pleasure package, but they're actually two distinct physiological phenomena that need not occur simultaneously. Train your guy how to separate one from the other, and he can have orgasms galore without setting loose his little swimmers, which is what typically pulls the plug on his hard-on and puts an end to the festivities. First, he needs to learn how to contract his pubococcygeal (or PC) muscle, which lines the pelvic cavity and can be located by stopping the flow of urine. Clenching this muscle can also halt the flow of seminal fluid from the body. Before he can do this he may need to build up his strength first by flexing these muscles twenty or more times per day for a week on his own. (If you're familiar with Kegel exercises, this is the male equivalent.)

Once you two are ready to give multiple Os a go together, start off by stimulating him as usual. The moment he feels that first flutter of orgasmic contractions, you should stop all stimulation while he squeezes his PC muscle as hard as he can. In doing so, he can prevent ejaculation while those orgasmic contractions keep flowing. He can repeat this pleasurable process as many times as he pleases, although eventually he'll probably want to top things off by busting loose with an orgasm/ejaculation finale.

6

MANUAL MOVES THAT WILL
ROCK HIS WORLD

Finally, here's where you learn how to use your hands on his Big Kahuna in ways that will make him gasp, "What was *that*? Can you do it again? Don't stop!" and other appreciative comments about the nature of your sexual genius. Men may have active imaginations about all the knee-buckling sensations their genitals could experience, but even so, your hands will be way ahead of them. The techniques you'll learn in this chapter make use of your palms, fingers, knuckles, and nails in surprising and creative combos. He won't know what hit him when you break out these moves.

Probably the best part is, unlike dabbling in backbreaking sex positions, expensive props, or complicated role-playing scenarios, you'll find that the techniques in this chapter all share one refreshingly common denominator: They're *easy*. Even our most complex maneuvers can be mastered in a few minutes, which can be a huge relief for couples who don't have the time to put on a big bells-and-whistles production in bed. Manual techniques are also highly compatible with other sexual activities. In chapter 10 we'll show you how to incorporate your handiwork into intercourse, oral sex, and other areas of your love life that could use some help. For now, though, let's let your hands take center stage and learn a few tricks that will amaze and astound.

COCK SHIATSU

Fine when he is erect or soft, with or without lubrication

This technique isn't a caress but rather a series of squeezes that will fire up nerves *underneath* the skin and boost circulation (and better blood flow = bigger erection). To start out, form a ring around the base of his penis with your thumb and middle finger. Tighten the ring for about one second, then release (try to exert most of the pressure on the sides of the penis versus front and back, since the front and back contain veins that might be painful if pinched too hard). Next move your "ring" up half an inch and squeeze again, continuing up the shaft and finishing off with one final squeeze on the head.

In addition to stimulating deeper tissue and getting the blood pumping, this technique also hits a series of acupressure points on the penis that are linked to other areas of the body. The head of the penis, or glans, for example, is connected to the pineal gland. The top third of the penis correlates to the spleen, mouth, stomach, and pancreas; the middle third to the liver, eyes, and small intestine; the bottom third near the base connects to the large intestines, kidney, and bladder. By squeezing these spots, you get energy spreading to all sorts of places. All in all, Cock Shiatsu is a powerful head-to-toe pick-me-up and a great way to launch a lusty encounter.

PENIS POWER STRETCH

Best when he is soft, without lubrication

Hold the head of the penis firmly in one hand and slowly pull—first down toward his feet, then to the sides, then up, then all around in a 360-degree circle, taking a full five seconds for each movement. While generally one doesn't think to stretch the penis like one would their hamstrings before running a 5K, the truth is, this exercise provides a unique—and highly pleasurable—sensation. Trust us, it won't hurt; penises live to lengthen. Just be sure to check in with your partner about how far is *too* far—although most times we hear men in our classes say, "Keep going!" Not only does this technique feel good; it has long-term benefits: You'll make his erections bigger, longer, and stronger. Permanently. We're not saying size is everything, but we think you'll find that most guys sure wouldn't complain if their minnow were a bit more like Moby Dick.

SHAKE, RATTLE, AND ROLL

Best when he is soft, without lubrication

Wrap your hand around the head of the penis and hold the penis straight out so that it is at a 90-degree angle to his body. Then move his penis in small circles like you were testing out the joystick on a video game. Start with five slow circles, then five fast, then (here's the clincher) give it a shake. That's right, shake that shaft as if you were playing the maracas in a mariachi band. Don't worry, his penis can handle it. Wiggling stimulates tissue in an entirely new way; aside from feeling good, it exudes tons of personality. It's playful and a perfect way to show him who's *really* in charge.

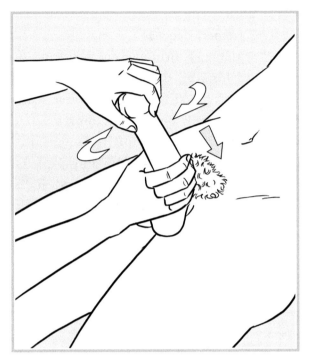

THE JUICER

THE JUICER

Best when he is erect, with lubrication

If you remember your anatomy lesson from chapter 5, you'll recall that the head of the penis, or glans, contains many more nerves than does the shaft. As a result it deserves some VIP treatment (and FYI, that *P* stands for *penis*). To deliver in spades, hold the base of the shaft with one hand and pull down. This will tug the skin at the head taut, which serves to further increase sensitivity by fully exposing those nerve endings.

Now that he's primed to feel even the subtlest sensations, take your other hand (lubricated is best) and loosely encase the head of his penis so that your fingers form a claw around it and your fingertips are encircling the corona. Twist your wrist in half circles, lightly stroking the head of his penis, making a motion as if you were juicing an orange.

TIGHT SQUEEZE

Best when he is erect, with lubrication

As with The Juicer, this technique lavishes attention on the extra-sensitive head of the penis. Only this time, rather than teasing him into a frenzy, you're going to lay it on thick and send him into sensory overload. Again, hold the base of the penis and pull down so the skin is taut. With the other hand (which should be well lubed), make a fist with a small opening . . . then slowly push the head of the penis through while squeezing tightly.

In case you haven't guessed, this technique mimics that extremely satisfying moment he enters other orifices in your body (such as the vagina or anus). And since your hand can adjust the tightness, the sensations you deliver can be *very* intense (just remember, the tighter your grip, the slower you should go to avoid overwhelming his nerve endings). Once you have inched your way past the head, continue sliding down the shaft and then move back on up. Then repeat to his heart's (or, rather, his hard-on's) content.

TWIST 'N' SHOUT

Best when he is erect, with lubrication

This technique is exactly the same as the Tight Squeeze, only you're adding a twist—literally. When your hand is wrapped around the head on either the down- or upstroke, torque your wrist and rotate your fist. This will further fire up his nerve endings and feel amazing.

RATTLE ON

Best when he is erect or semierect, with or without lubrication

Cup your hand loosely over the head of the penis in a claw shape. Then quickly jiggle your hand so that the head bounces around against your fingers in the space below. This cheeky move can be a refreshing break after you have been doing a lot of smooth stroking. It injects the element of surprise, which will only fuel the excitement.

LOOP DE LOOP

Fine when he is erect or soft, best with lubrication

Take your thumb and forefinger and form a loop or ring like an "OK" sign. Wrap this ring around the corona—the ridge where the head meets the shaft. Lightly inch up and down so you're massaging right over the lip. Since so many nerve endings lie along this loop, the slightest movement here will trigger intense pleasure and convince him you've got the magic touch.

TICKLE THE PICKLE

Fine when he is erect or soft, best with lubrication

The frenulum, you may recall, is an extra-sensitive spot on the underside of the coronal ridge where the head meets the shaft. Even tiny movements here can produce huge results, and this technique fits the bill to a tee. Place both thumbs on the underside of the corona and find a comfortable way to rest your hands—either on his stomach if he's lying down, or cradling the shaft of his penis if he's standing up. Then using both thumbs start massaging dime-sized circles right on the frenulum.

TRICKS TO TRY IF HE'S UNCIRCUMCISED

If your fella has never had his foreskin snipped, that means there's even *more* penis to play with! The main thing to know about this extra layer of skin covering the glans is that you can actually move it up and down (especially when the penis is soft or semierect). What's more, the motion itself can create tons of feel-good friction. Here's how to use this info to your (and his) advantage:

PEEKABOO
Can be done when he is soft to semierect, with or without lubrication
Wrap your hand around the foreskin, which should still be covering the head of the penis, then shimmy the entire foreskin up and down so you're essentially playing peekaboo with the head. This will stimulate two supersensitive areas—the foreskin and the glans underneath—for twice the sensory overload.

TICKLING THE TURTLENECK
Can be done when he is soft to semierect, with or without lubrication
Hold the head of the penis between thumb and fingers with your fingers on the side facing his stomach. Rub your thumb over the frenulum (a spot right under the glans on the side facing out) so you're inching the foreskin up and down over that area. As with Peekaboo, you're turning on two areas at once: the foreskin and the frenulum. It's multitasking at its finest.

Once an uncircumcised penis gains steam and the foreskin retracts, it should largely look and feel like circumcised models and can be treated as such. Still, this will vary from guy to guy, so be sure to check in and make sure he's enjoying himself.

V FOR VICTORY

Best when he is erect, lubrication a must

With the index and middle finger of both hands in a V shape, close them around his penis so that the crooks between your fingers are hugging the shaft. Then slide your hands up and down. The smooth sides of your fingers will feel refreshingly different from your more textured palm and fingertips. Switch back and forth between the two types of sensations to spark new life into his nerve endings.

GETTING IT FROM BOTH ENDS

Best when he is erect, with lubrication

For this move, you'll want him lying on his back with his penis resting on his stomach. Using thumb and forefinger, gently squeeze the tissue at the base of the shaft closest to his belly and push down slightly. This should make the shaft rise a bit from its position of repose and angle up toward the ceiling. Then, keeping your pinch hold, knead the base of the penis in tiny circles, which will stimulate blood flow into the shaft and create an even firmer erection.

Meanwhile, take the thumb and forefinger of your other hand, form a ring like an "OK" sign, wrap it around the corona, and lightly stroke up and down so you're massaging right over the ridge. Combined, these two moves can send men into overdrive because not only are you targeting two very sensitive areas—the corona and the base—but you're stimulating them in different *ways*. Up top he'll enjoy some feathery stroking, while down below you're providing a contrast with an invigorating pinch-and-pull. This technique will require a little concentration, but you'll be glad you made the effort.

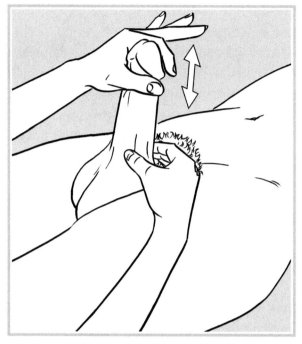

GETTING IT FROM BOTH ENDS

L FOR LUST

Best when he is erect, lubrication a must

Hold your thumbs and index fingers out at right angles to each other as if you were creating an L. Then place your Ls on each side of the penis and move them up and down so that the webbing between thumb and forefinger is gently grazing the shaft. No area of your hand can deliver as soft and velvety a sensation—in fact, it might feel strikingly similar to another soft, velvety area of a woman's anatomy (hello, vagina) and convince him of just how talented your hands truly are.

THE SIDEWINDER

Best when he is erect, lots of lubrication a must

Once you are ready to *really* heat things up, flatten your hands and place them on the sides of the shaft parallel to each other. Start sliding your hands in opposing directions—one up while the other goes down, then back the other way—as if you were rolling Play-Doh between your palms to make a snake. Keep your hands moving in this manner as you shift them slowly up and down the shaft. This technique stimulates his nerve endings in an entirely new direction (sideways versus up and down) and creates a *lot* of friction that is bound to stoke his coals.

THE SIDEWINDER II

Best when he is erect, lots of lubrication a must

One variation of The Sidewinder entails not keeping your hands flat but wrapping them around the shaft and twisting in opposite directions. This creates even *more* feel-good friction than the original move. Just make sure you use lots of lubrication and don't squeeze too hard, or it might be too much stimulation for one guy to handle.

SCRATCHING POST

Best when he is erect, fine with or without lubrication

This technique gets your nails in on the action. Lightly stroke the shaft of the penis with just the tips of your talons, trying your best to avoid rubbing your fingertips along the shaft as well. The tiny pinpricks your nails provide will give him chills—and don't worry, if you do this lightly, he'll be moaning in pleasure rather than pain.

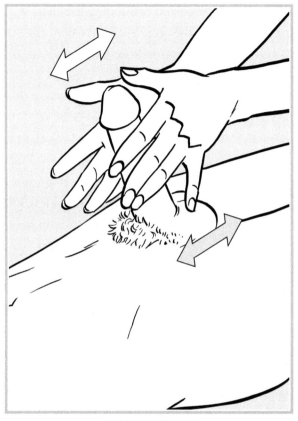

THE SIDEWINDER

SCRATCHING POST IN REVERSE

Best when he is erect, fine with or without lubrication

If your nails are too short to pull off the Scratching Post technique without your fingertips getting in the way, try this alternative. Rub the shaft of his penis with the *backs* of your talons. You can use just the tips of the backs of your nails for a sharper sensation, or curl your fingers under a little more so you're rubbing the shaft with the entire flat of your nails and even the cuticles. Either way, the sensation will be a novelty your partner is sure to appreciate.

PAVLOV'S PENIS

Fine when he is erect or soft, with or without lubrication

Chances are you've all heard the story of Pavlov's dog, where some pooch was trained to associate the sound of a bell with snack time and drool on command. We're not saying men are dogs, but this type of psychological conditioning can work in bed, too. Here's how: Covering your hands with massage oil, place one hand on his genitals and the other in the center of his chest. Keeping your hands flat and relaxed, start massaging small circles on both areas.

In effect, you're stimulating his sexuality (in his genitals) and his sentimental side (in his heart). Done simultaneously, this technique will cultivate a link between love and lust and get him to subconsciously associate urges like *I'm horny* with thoughts like *I'm totally in love with this person.* If it's more romance you crave in the sack, this move may do the trick.

PATTY CAKE

Best when he is erect, with or without lubrication

Flatten your hands, take the penis between them, then start gently slapping it back and forth from palm to palm. Sure, this technique might seem like some kind of cruel joke at first, but it can feel wonderfully invigorating and increase circulation to the surface of the skin, further increasing sensitivity. So go ahead, bandy that boner around and see what he thinks.

TUMMY RUB

Fine when he is erect or soft, best with lots of lubrication

With your partner lying faceup, drip some warm lubrication or massage oil below his belly button, then rest his penis there. Placing the heel of your hand firmly against the shaft, start moving the penis back and forth across his stomach like a windshield wiper. Since he's probably never received a "tummy job" before, the novelty alone will win you originality points. Plus, whether it's a six-pack or a paunch, hairy or smooth, the contact of his penis with his abdomen will provide a unique sensation he's bound to appreciate. Finally, let's not forget that you're also stimulating his stomach, which, according to Tantric traditions, is the center of his sense of power.

GREAT BALLS OF FIRE

Best with lubrication

The oft-ignored testicles are two jewels just waiting to be plundered, yet if you're a little shaky on how to handle his *huevos*, here's a great way to get started. Encircle the base of the testicles between thumb and index finger, then gently pull them away from the body so you're holding them in a compact sack. This will stretch the skin taut, exposing more nerve endings and upping his sensitivity levels to lofty new heights. Start lightly stroking the scrotum with the fingertips of your other hand, or tickling with your nails, or alternating between the two. The effects will feel electric—and there are other benefits. Pulling the testicles away from the body tends to pull him back from the brink if he's about to blow (more on that next).

WHOA NELLY

Best when he is erect, with lubrication

If he's approaching his big finale but you aren't ready to call it a night, this move will put on the brakes, but in a pleasurable way. With both hands wrapped around his penis one stacked on top of the other, move the top hand toward the head of his penis and the other down toward his testicles so that you're essentially pulling up on the penis with one hand and down toward the testicles with the other. Hold for a beat, then release and repeat. In chapter 5 we described how prior to ejaculation, the testicles rise a bit toward the body; by pulling down on them, you relax the area and keep things in check. Meanwhile, your other upward-moving hand will keep him sufficiently stimulated to stay in this holding pattern.

SCROTUM YOGA

Best without lubrication

Ever see those dudes on TV who hang huge weights from their nuts? Call them crazy, but the truth is, testicles *like* to be stretched. We're not saying you should chain andirons to your guy's juju's any time soon, but he may find this scaled-down exercise extremely satisfying. Using thumb and forefinger, gently get a pinch hold of the scrotal sack right between the testicles where the skin is loosest. Gingerly pull the skin down toward his feet. If that makes him happy, try pulling forward, then back, or slowly swinging the skin back and forth like a pendulum. Remember to check in with him here; he may want more stretch than you imagined. As long as you don't twist, the sensation should feel pretty damn good—and you should be cured of the silly notion that his eggs are too delicate to deal with.

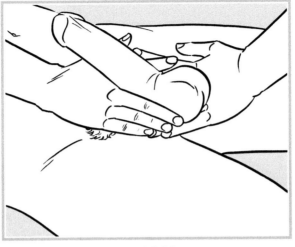

THE ROOT

THE ROOT

Fine when he is erect or soft, best with lubrication

Raise your index and middle fingers in a V shape and wedge one V under the testicles so that the crook between your fingers is touching the perineum, that extra-sensitive patch of skin behind the testicles. Meanwhile, wedge the other V on the top side of the base of the penis so that the palm of that hand is resting against his stomach. Slowly bring your two Vs toward one another as close as they'll get (depending on the length of your fingers and the size of his package, your fingertips might touch or even cross at the ends).

Once your Vs are in position, start inching them up and down, back and forth, or in tiny circles, keeping your movements small as the Vs hug the base. While this technique might not seem to offer much in the stimulation department, that's only because the action is

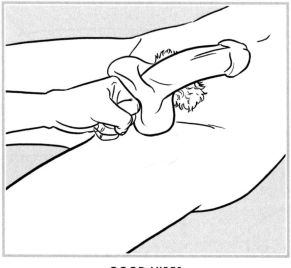

GOOD VIBES

occurring deep within the *root* of his penis, testicles, and perineum. As long as *he* feels it, you're doing fine.

GOOD VIBES

Fine when he is erect or soft, with or without lubrication

This technique requires a little participation on his part—namely, he moans while it's being done. Maybe he'll be moaning anyway (so no problem there), but if not, ask him to give it a try so he can feel the full effects. To start, make a fist with one hand. Without bending your wrist, place your fist up against his perineum, the area between his testicles and his anus. Begin vibrating your fist back and forth, which will stimulate his perineum and the extra-sensitive prostate gland underneath.

At this point, ask him to start moaning or humming—anything that will get his vocal chords working will do. This vocalizing will help the tremors from below travel up from his perineum, through his prostate, and even further. In essence, his entire torso will be able to feel the buzz. The sensation is so unique that he probably won't be able to explain what it's like, other than to say, "Wow, cool. Keep doing it."

7

HOW TO GIVE HER A HAND

SAMANTHA: Is he really that bad in bed?

MIRANDA: No, he's just . . . he's a guy. They can rebuild a jet engine but when it comes to a woman, what's the big mystery? It's my clitoris, not the Sphinx.

—*SEX AND THE CITY*

Admit it: No matter how many times you've been graced with its presence, a woman's genital region can be far from easy to figure out. Sometimes nothing under the sun seems to steer a woman toward liftoff, and while women may kvetch about your cluelessness, oftentimes *they* don't know what will work either (or, if they do know, they aren't forthcoming enough to explain). It's no wonder many of us spend more time scratching our heads than striking gold.

And yet, for all its intricacies, Pandora's box *can* be unlocked—

and pretty easily, provided you learn a few key things. Peruse this chapter and all will be illuminated. Some women have trouble reaching orgasm and may want to do so more consistently. Others may have no trouble reaching climax but may want to experience multiple peaks. Still others may want to embark on a quest for their G-spot and try ejaculating. Whatever your goal, don't get frustrated if you don't immediately figure it out (haven't you ever heard it's the journey that counts?). Follow the pointers in this chapter and you'll definitely be heading down the right path.

First, let's take a peek beneath those bikini briefs and behold her in all her glory. Knowing her genital area's various components is essential if you want to start tinkering, and this is one user's manual we highly doubt you'll mind reading.

HER VA-NATOMY, EXPLAINED

Perhaps the number one reason people are often in the dark about women's genitals is that their owners aren't always all that enthusiastic about showing them off. Unlike men, who are largely at peace with the appearance of their penis and would probably love nothing more than to have someone gaze at it longingly, women are often conditioned to think that the less attention that area "down there" gets, the better. Even uttering the word "vagina" makes some women squirm and resort to euphemisms. That said, while some women may be reluctant to formally introduce you to their privates and various parts, we'd be happy to show you around.

Many people call the whole kit and caboodle "the vagina," but the visible area in its entirety is actually called the *vulva*. Now that we've cleared that up, let's examine some of its assorted features.

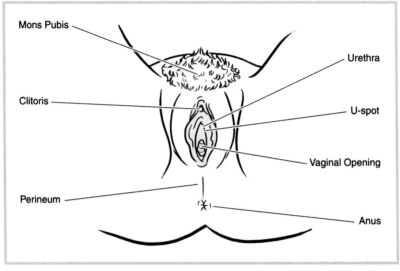

THE FEMALE GENITALS

The Mons Pubis

This cushiony mound right above her main attractions may be covered in pubic hair or waxed smooth. Either way, while people often skate right past because of their eagerness to explore more exciting environs, the mons pubis (or mons for short) is a major destination unto itself. Given that it surrounds some extremely sensitive areas below, merely cupping this hillock and jiggling it or drumming your fingers on the top can warm up more nerve endings than you'd ever imagine. All in all, it's well worth your time to linger here a little.

The Clitoris

Located below the mons pubis at the crest of the vaginal opening, this little love button is packed with eight thousand nerve endings—that's

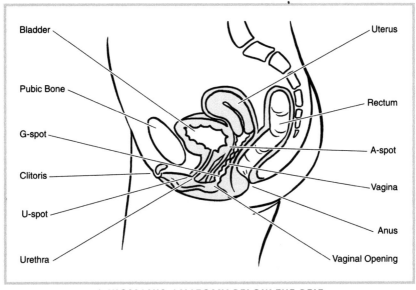

A WOMAN'S ANATOMY BELOW THE BELT

twice as many as the entire penis contains (read it and weep, fellahs). As a result, this tiny kernel can trigger hoards of pleasure, although it should definitely be handled with care. Many women may find direct stimulation here too overwhelming (especially during the initial stages of foreplay), so tread lightly at first and see how she reacts.

For many women, the clitoris remains tucked away under the *clitoral hood* or *prepuce*. Like the top on a convertible, though, this layer of skin can be pulled back if you press up on the mons, revealing the pink nub that's the sexual center of a woman's universe. While the clitoris may seem small (especially compared to a man's package), there's much more to it than meets the eye. Similar to a penis, a clitoris contains erectile tissue, gets larger when aroused, and is composed of a head (or *glans*) and shaft, each of which can be stimulated with some finesse. What's more, keep in mind that all you're seeing is the *visible* portion of the clitoris; the rest of it extends three to four inches beneath the skin. All in all, the clitoris is full of surprises and should never be underestimated.

The Labia

Surrounding the vaginal opening are some folds of skin otherwise known as the labia, and there are actually two sets adorning this entrance. The outer set, or *labia majora,* are covered with pubic hair (unless she waxes or shaves). Between those lie the *labia minora,* which will swell in size and can change color from pink to purple when the excitement builds. While many people view the labia purely as a curtained gateway to their final destination, the labia are actually very sensitive and deserve some attention in their own right. In the next chapter we will show you how to gently stroke, pinch, or even slowly pull them with fantastic results.

The Vagina

This area probably needs no introduction, and many of you would happily hang out here all day. Still, have you taken the time to *really* learn what's going on in there? Allow us to fill you in. For starters, every vagina is different. Some are shorter, others longer, some tighter, others roomier. What's more, while the *entire* vagina probably feels pretty darn good to you, to her, certain spots are much more sensitive than others. For most women, the area most worthy of attention lies along the front wall facing her stomach. Your hands are perfectly designed to do this area justice. We'll explain how in more detail later, but here's a hint: Just insert a finger and move it in a come-hither motion against the front wall, which is home to the next two not-to-be-missed moan zones on our list—the G-spot and A-spot.

The G-spot

Named after Ernst Gräfenberg, a German doctor who first documented this area's existence in 1950, the G-spot is a quarter-sized rough patch lying on the front wall of the vagina one to three inches in. It is considered the equivalent of a man's prostate gland, a well-known erogenous zone. The sensitivity of the G-spot varies from woman to woman. Move your finger here in a come-hither motion, and some women will shrug and say they don't get it; others will hit the ceiling. In 1982 a study of four hundred women by sex researcher Beverly Whipple and her colleagues found that stimulating the G-spot could result in an orgasm—and not just any old orgasm, but one that causes women to ejaculate.

If you've witnessed a woman gush like Mount Vesuvius and wondered what the heck was going on, keep in mind that this mixture (which could amount to from a teaspoon to a few tablespoons) is definitely not urine but a mixture of glucose, fructose, proteins, and water (strangely, the fluid's origins are unknown, although the prevailing theory is that it is produced by the Skenes gland, which is located around the bottom part of the urethra). If you haven't seen a woman ejaculate but would like to, in the next chapter we'll provide plenty of advice on how to make her cup runneth over.

The A-spot

Also on the front wall of the vagina but three to four inches in lies another rough patch that might feel similar to the G-spot but is more spread out and bell-shaped. This is the anterior fornix erogenous zone, or A-spot for short. Theorized to be an extension of the G-spot, the A-spot was discovered in 1993 by Malaysian sex researcher Chua Chee Ann. His studies found that stimulating this area (a come-hither finger wiggle also works well here) can cause women to become lubricated in five to ten seconds, to become orgasmic in one to two minutes, and also can help women to ejaculate.

The U-spot

So named since it lies on top and/or to the sides of the urethral opening (which is right above the vagina), the U-spot not only is rich in nerve endings but contains another passion-inducing perk: erectile tissue. While the area is way too small to pop a noticeable hard-on, you might be able to feel a tiny bump with a fingertip after lightly tickling the area. And, as with the G-spot and A-spot, you might be able to get her to ejaculate by stimulating the U-spot.

The Perineum

This patch of skin between the vagina and the anus (aka "the taint" since " 'tain't one or the other") is a crossroads of nerve endings and muscle groups that are responsible for revving up the entire pelvic region. These muscle groups include the bulbocavernosis muscles (which assist in tightening the vaginal canal and creating a clitoral erection), the ischiocavernosus muscles (responsible for maintaining a clitoral erection), and others. Pressing on the perineum is like flooring the gas pedal on a Ferrari—it's bound to leave her breathless.

The Anus

If they could, many women would board off this area with a huge KEEP OUT sign spanning from cheek to cheek. If the woman you're with is one of these, that's her prerogative—it's her anus, after all. Still, the fact of the matter is, the anus contains more nerve endings than any other part of the body, second only to the genitals. So if she's into your exploring the area (and you're game to go there), turn to chapter 9 for details.

HANDLING HER ULTIMATE HOT SPOT: SOME GUIDELINES TO KEEP IN MIND

Now that you've got a good working knowledge of what's going on under the hood, let's bring your hands into the picture. In the next chapter we'll show you specific techniques that will rev her engines, but in the meantime here's some general advice that will help you avoid some common fumbles.

We Repeat: Your Finger Is Not a Penis

We know you know this, and yet time and again we see people (men *and* women) moving their hand in and out of the vagina in a thrusting motion that mimics *exactly* what a penis does down there to a tee. We're not saying this motion doesn't feel good or won't come in handy on certain occasions, but the whole point of using your hands is that they can do things a penis cannot. For instance, as we mentioned already, some of the vagina's most sensitive spots (such as the G-spot and A-spot) lie on its front wall a few inches in. The best way to stimulate these spots is not by chugging in and out like a piston, but by inserting a finger, holding it steady, and crooking it toward you in a come-hither motion so you're actually moving the tissue inside rather than just rubbing along its surface. This is just one of many ways your hands trump a hard-on in the stimulation department, so make sure to use your mitts to *their* full potential rather than treating them like a surrogate schlong.

Wash Your Hands Before They Wander

You know how moms always tell you to wash your hands before you eat? We'd like to add an addendum to that rule that we're sure few mothers would dare to mention: You should also wash your hands before you hop in the sack. It's a scientific fact that in any given day your hands come in contact with countless surfaces that are crawling with badass microorganisms. What's more, these germs most easily enter the body via the mucous membranes, which include the eyes, nose, mouth, and (last but not least) her vagina. Skip the soap and water and you could risk passing along anything from your garden-variety cold to the bacteria that cause a urinary tract infection, neither of which will do much for your sex life. Also keep in mind that bacteria often hide underneath fingernails, so make sure your nails are trimmed. For extra points, file them to avoid scraping any sharp edges across her delicate petals (ouch).

Take a Bathroom Break Before You Begin

This holds true for both genders, but women have added reason to hit the john before the games begin. As we mentioned earlier, stimulation of the G-spot, A-spot, or U-spot may prompt women to ejaculate—yet many women block this sensation since it feels strikingly similar to the need to pee. If she relieves herself ahead of time, however, she'll know that any calls of nature she gets in the midst of it all are probably fake, and that what's *really* happening is you've just hit an extra-sensitive area that could soon get her gushing.

Sex and Drugs Don't Mix

One glass of wine might help her unwind, but a few Long Island Iced Teas will get her bombed, not turned on. Not only does alcohol numb the nerves; it's also a diuretic that will desiccate her body's natural water supply—including the reserves she's got down below. Of course, you can use store-bought lubricant, but she won't appreciate your handiwork half as much if she's sloshed. Also keep in mind that certain prescription medications—such as antidepressants—can cause numbness and make orgasm difficult. If she thinks her meds are cramping the fun, she can talk to her doctor about switching to ones with fewer sexual side effects.

Sweet-talk Her Sweet Spot

As silly as it sounds, many women are worried their vaginas look, smell, or taste funny. And this self-consciousness can keep her from enjoying all the attention you're lavishing down there. To ease her embarrassment, pay her privates a compliment. A simple "It's beautiful" or "I love the way you smell/taste/feel" will perk up her sexual self-confidence and her satisfaction levels as well.

Request a Hands-on Demonstration

It's simple: Nobody knows how to play her pipe organs like she does. So if you *really* want to learn how and where she likes to be touched, watching her masturbate will be your best tutorial ever. We're not saying you should sit there and take notes; rather, treat it like a feast for the eyes by telling her what a turn-on it is to see her pleasure herself. If she's too shy to put on a show, she might feel less self-conscious if you *both* masturbate in front of each other. Another alternative is to put your hands on her privates then ask her to place her hands on top of yours and move them the way she likes. No matter how you conduct class, you're bound to learn by example.

This Delicate Tulip Is Actually Anything But

While it's true you'll want to treat the ultra-sensitive clitoris with care and tread lightly there, the rest of a woman's genitals are actually much sturdier than you might think. Many of the techniques we teach in the next chapter require that you pinch, slap, and stretch things in ways that might first make you wonder *Whoa, won't that hurt?* But in our experience, people more often err on the side of using too light or tentative a touch—and the effects can feel irritating rather than arousing, like an itch she wants to scratch. So don't be afraid to handle her vulva with confidence. For additional guidance, ask, "Does that hurt or do you want me to keep going?" and adjust your touch accordingly.

Don't Rush It

A woman's motor often takes time to warm up—which is probably why the most common mistake people make is to try to move things along at too quick a clip. No matter how slow you're going, go more slowly. Think like a painter and make every stroke count. Your goal is not so much to give her an orgasm but to allow her orgasm to come to you. To make sure you proceed at her pace, ask for her feedback, or take cues from her body language: If her hips seem to be pulling away you're coming on too strong; if they rise to meet you consider that a green light.

Ask Before You Enter

Think about it: Before you enter a room, it's only polite to knock. Same goes with the vagina. Given that people tend to rush things, it can help to have an extra safeguard that'll keep you from barging in before she's game for guests. While asking, "Are you ready for me to enter you?" is a good start, she may feel obligated to say yes. So instead offer her a choice by asking, "Are you ready for me to enter you or would you rather I continue teasing you?" That way she is allowed to choose rather than refuse what you're offering, and things can continue on a positive note.

Don't Fret If She's Not Wet

You're pulling out all the stops, yet yonder valleys remain devoid of their usual dewiness. That means she's bored out of her mind, right? Not necessarily. A woman's natural lubrication levels ebb and flow due to all sorts of factors, from medication she's taking to where she's at in her menstrual cycle. Therefore using wetness as a gauge to assess her state of arousal is not always reliable. So here's your reality check: If she's wet, she's wet. If she's dry, don't take it personally; go grab that tube of lube you've got stashed in your nightstand.

It's Okay If She's Not Shouting in Ecstasy

While porn videos sure make it seem as if all women screech at the top of their lungs during sex, the reality is, everyone expresses their pleasure differently. A choice few may be screamers; others may only quiver and sigh. Some may start tearing their (and your) hair out; others will largely lie there and not move an inch. So don't assume your efforts aren't appreciated if she's barely making a peep. When in doubt, ask. Your interest shows you care (which will shine well on you no matter what). From there, she can either steer you in a better direction or reassure you that she's having a ball.

Experiment with Different Positions

If you thought that there was only *one* position in which to manually stimulate her genitals (her on her back and you lying within arm's reach), that's not the half of it. There are plenty of alternatives, and even small adjustments in body position can make a big difference arousal-wise. Consider these options:

- Her lying on her back with her legs raised, knees or feet resting on your shoulders while you sit on the mattress below her butt with your legs spread in a V to each side of her body. This twist offers some tantalizing access to rear-end attractions like her perineum and anus.

- Her lying on her back with her hips near the edge of the bed, you kneeling on the floor. Since your head and torso can remain vertical as you work your magic, you can avoid neck and shoulder strain.

- Her lying on her side, you spooning her from behind or lying face-to-face—a prime choice for those of you who crave plenty of eye contact and kissing.

- Her on all fours, you kneeling or standing behind her—a highly erotic, animalistic pose that also offers great access to all her backside has to offer.

- Her standing, legs slightly spread or with one leg up on a chair or the bed, you kneeling beneath. Her sense of power will soar as you aim to please from down under.

Leverage Her Legs to Your Advantage

Raised or lowered, together or apart, leg position is pivotal to her pleasure. Whatever technique you're trying, its success may hinge on where her limbs are located. Move them around, and you may be surprised to find certain angles will get her singing your praises louder than others. While each woman will have her own personal preferences, here's what you can expect in general:

- If she's on her back and her legs are raised, this tends to pitch the angle of her vagina upward, making it easier to stimulate the G-spot and A-spot during manual stimulation, intercourse, or otherwise.
- If her legs are apart, this gives you better access to all her nooks and crannies (obviously).
- If her legs are together, this may limit access somewhat, but there are definite benefits. Given everything's situated snugly together, you can stimulate *more* real estate with every stroke.
- If one leg is up and the other down, you'll get the best of both worlds: better access, but also tons of feel-good friction.

Watch What You're Doing

Granted your sense of touch will take you far in terms of finding and rousing her erogenous zones. That said, whenever possible it sure can't hurt to eyeball things a little. The clitoris, for one, can be hard to find unless you pull back the clitoral hood and scrutinize the area for the telltale pink nub. And you're flying totally blind on the U-spot unless you spread the inner labia and search for a tiny hole (that's the urethra where the U-spot is located). It can also help to have a visual sense of how her genitals change throughout the arousal process. The clitoris may become larger and/or more pronounced, her inner labia may change color from pink to purple. Know the signs and you can more accurately gauge whether she's still warming up or ready to blow. Of course, we're not suggesting you shine a spotlight here as if you were conducting a gyno exam, but whatever visuals you can gather will only work in your favor.

Don't Get Too Caught Up in Doing It "Right"

Can't quite get the knack of that finger wiggle technique? Don't sweat it. Focus to a fault, and you will be distracted from your ultimate goal, which is to make sure *she's* having fun. And we mean *all* of her, not just that small patch between her legs. To maintain intimacy levels, tear your eyes away from the prize occasionally and engage in some cuddling above the belt. Do that and chances are she won't care if your execution of some of our maneuvers isn't perfect. In fact, she may like your version better since it comes from her favorite person: you.

Found a Technique She Loves? Great—Now Move On

Congratulations, you've discovered that Bowing the Violin gets her reeling in ecstasy. Take note, then go try something else. While a woman's anatomy is often so tricky it's tempting to stick with what works, setting Bowing the Violin on repeat won't exactly impress. The genitals crave variety, and given all the techniques there are to explore in this book, you might be surprised to find before the evening is done that there are many others she adores. And even if nothing lights her fire quite like Bowing, you'll have fun trying, and you can always turn back to your old reliable any time to bring on orgasmic bliss.

Make Sure She Breathes Deeply

When arousal builds, many women react by tensing their bodies and holding their breath. This impulse actually holds women back. Not only is breathing important in helping your partner relax and really let go, but when the body is excited, nerve endings need oxygen—lots of it—to process pleasurable sensations. So make sure she's inhaling and exhaling deep into her belly. This will shuttle more oxygen-rich blood into her pelvis, and make your every hands-on move feel even more amazing.

Don't Call It Quits After One Climax

Women's genitals are blessed with a short refractory period, which means that even if she's just had an orgasm, she can turn right around and have another . . . and another. Since that's the case, why stop at just one? After laying off on all stimulation for a few seconds to let her recover from Big O #1, start warming her up again. Most women may be sensitive at this point, so start off with light strokes or move to a less-trafficked erogenous zone like her labia or her nipples before you transition to more intense, tried-and-true orgasm-inducing techniques. Remind her to breathe deeply and ask her for direction on what she'd like you to do, and you may both be surprised how quickly Big O #2, #3, and more arrive on the scene.

Don't Freak If She Doesn't Reach Her Peak

Sometimes, no matter what you do, an orgasm just isn't in the cards. And while determination pays off in many areas of life from landing a promotion to completing a 5K race, with orgasms the opposite is true: Sometimes, the harder you try, the more elusive they become. We're not saying you should call it quits after five minutes, but if you've been going at it for a while and have a hunch you've reached a sexual stalemate, ask her if there's anything you could do to turn things around. She may have some ideas, or she may just tell you to throw in the towel. Whatever the case, don't beat yourself up about it. Remember that orgasm or no, most women find physical intimacy rewarding in its own right.

Ease Out of Sex Slowly

Whether you've whipped up a triple-whammy orgasm extravaganza or things culminated on a less climactic note, what you do during the dénouement is important, too. After sex a woman's body starts producing a chemical called oxytocin—nicknamed the "cuddle chemical" since it prompts women to do just that. Given her mental state, probably the *worst* thing you could do at this point is to abruptly withdraw, roll over, and call it a night. Instead maintain the connection by wrapping your arms around her, or holding hands, or cupping your palm over her vulva. Say something sweet like "you're amazing" or, if that's too over the top given the circumstances, comment on the experience itself by saying, "That was amazing," or even a simple "Wow" will suffice. We're not saying you need to stay entwined in each other's arms all night if that's not your cup of tea, but as far as we're concerned, a little postcoital contact adds the perfect finishing touch.

8

MANUAL MOVES THAT WILL
ROCK HER WORLD

Prepare to knock your lady's knickers off. In this chapter we're going to open your eyes to all the amazing things your hands can do that may whip her into a hair-wrenching, sheet-drenching frenzy. Whether the woman you're with has trouble reaching her peak or just wants longer, stronger, or just plain more *Oh-my-god* moments, this bag of tricks has all your bases covered. In fact, given the constellation of trigger points she's got below the belt, there are actually *more* techniques to try on a woman's anatomy than on a man's (sorry, fellahs, them's the breaks).

What's more, it bears repeating that you can use these techniques not only during foreplay but also *during* intercourse, oral sex, and other mattress antics that you've come to love. Learn how to weave your handiwork into every facet of your sex life (we'll show you how in chapter 10), and don't be surprised if you see her libido skyrocket. Because the truth is, given that the layout of a woman's nether regions is far from straightforward, using your hands isn't just a nice touch, it's a *necessity*. Learn how to use them to their full potential, and you will unleash *her* full potential to adore and crave sex. Think that sounds worth the effort? Try a few of these tricks then watch what happens.

VULVA YOGA
Best without lubrication

While many think that the only way to handle a woman's privates is to rub them, that's not the half of it—and here's a great way to start expanding your horizons. Using both hands, squeeze the sides of her outer labia (the fleshy areas to each side of her vagina) between thumb and forefinger and gradually stretch them toward her feet. This technique tends to frighten people at first and make them wonder *Can I really do that?* We can confidently say that on some women you can pull pretty darn hard (although you'll want to check in with her to make sure it's not *too* much).

Chances are she's never had her vulva stretched before, so not only do you have the element of surprise on your side, but the sensation feels wonderful—relaxing, invigorating, and a little racy all at once (plus it boosts blood flow to the area, which will further increase sensitivity). If a downward pull gets rave reviews, try pulling the outer labia up, to the sides, or stretching one up and one down.

THE WAVE
Fine with or without lubrication

This one starts simple: Cup the entire vulva with your hand, with the heel of your palm resting on the mons (where her pubic bone is) and your fingers extending southward over the inner and outer labia. In itself, cupping the vulva can feel very comforting, and can be a sweet way to start or end any sex session. That said, what you're about to do next will amp things up.

Remember back in the eighties when a dance move called The Wave was all the rage? Even if that was before your time, we're sure you can imagine what it looks like: Still cupping the vulva, start undulating your hand, pressing first on the mons with the heel of your hand, then the clitoris with the upper palm, then the labia with your fingers, and so on, over and over. While a woman might at first wonder what the heck you're doing, she'll soon change her tune once she feels the effects, which can fire up the entire region—mons, clitoris, labia, vagina—in one fell swoop.

LITTLE EARTHQUAKE
Fine with or without lubrication
Rest the heel of your hand an inch or so above her pubic bone so that your curled fingers rest comfortably on the crest of her mons pubis. Then start tapping or drumming your fingers lightly on the area. This will send reverberations throughout the vulva and even wake up nerve endings underneath the skin. All in all, it's a great way to get the entire area buzzing.

SHAKEN NOT STIRRED
Fine with or without lubrication
Cup your hand over the vulva as you did with The Wave. Only this time press down firmly and jiggle your hand, as well as everything underneath it. Do this fast enough, and the effects may feel similar to that of a vibrator and trigger some pretty sexy results.

BOWING THE VIOLIN

Best with lots of lubrication

There are a variety of ways to touch a woman's clitoris, and this one is a show stopper. Treat your index or middle finger like the bow of a violin, sliding the entire front side of the finger over the clitoris from tip to base. You can glide so lightly that you're barely touching, or add more pressure for more of a climactic crescendo.

ROCK AROUND THE CLIT

Best with lots of lubrication

We don't need to tell you that the clitoris is extremely sensitive, but what you might *not* know is that certain parts are more sensitive than others. To find your partner's own personal sweet spot, envision a tiny clock face on top of the clitoris, then rub on the hour, every hour. This can be tough since the area is small, but allow yourself to enjoy the time it takes to be precise. And if you closely gauge her reaction at each stop, you may come away knowing exactly what "time" you should tend to most. Strange, but true: Two o'clock seems to be the most popular Happy Hour among women. We don't know why, but it has proven true in almost every class we teach.

JILLING OFF

Best with lots of lubrication

While people generally think of "jacking off" solely as a man's prerogative, the clitoris, while small, does have a shaft—and with some finesse it can be stroked in a similar way. To find the shaft, push up on the mons to expose the clitoris, then start feeling around for a firm stalk extending beneath the pink nub of the clitoral head. Once you've located the shaft, gently pinch it between thumb and forefinger and

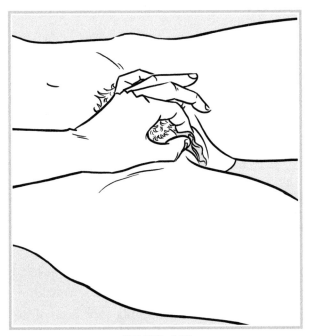

JILLING OFF

massage this tiny clit boner up and down. Keep in mind, every millimeter you move hits thousands of nerve endings, so even if your actions seem almost microscopic, you'll still trigger hair-raising results.

KNUCKLE SANDWICH

Best with lots of lubrication

If you've mastered Jilling Off and can easily locate the shaft of the clitoris, try this alternative: Pinch the shaft between the knuckles of your index and middle finger, then stroke up and down so that the sides of your knuckles are rubbing the shaft of the clitoris. Try experimenting with different speeds and pressures.

TUNING IN

Best with lots of lubrication

This technique also requires that you locate the clitoral shaft (for more details, see Jilling Off). Gently squeeze the shaft between thumb and forefinger as in Jilling Off, only rather than stroking up and down, rotate your fingers back and forth as if you were adjusting a dial. This will stimulate the shaft in a sideways direction versus up and down; this technique is often even easier to accomplish than Jilling Off, especially if her clitoris is small.

RINGING THE DOORBELL

Fine with or without lubrication

Using the pad of your thumb, press firmly against the head of the clitoris and hold for a count of four. Then release your thumb quickly and repeat. This technique won't stimulate the head of the clitoris so much as it will turn on the shaft, which will be forced to contract under the pressure—you might even feel it dance under your thumb as it resists. By releasing your touch quickly, you bring blood rushing back into the area and make this little love button spring back to life, stronger and more sensitive than ever.

KNOCKING ON HEAVEN'S DOOR

Fine with or without lubrication

Once the clitoris is fully aroused and your partner is on the brink of a Big O, this technique can help you linger on this delicious precipice indefinitely. Using the tip of your index finger, gently tap-tap-tap on the head of the clitoris. This teasing touch provides just enough stimulation to keep her aroused, but not enough to send her over the edge.

U-TURN

Best with lubrication

If you did due diligence and read up on her below-the-belt anatomy in chapter 7, you'll recall that below the clitoris and above the vagina lies a little-known erogenous zone called the U-spot, so named because it lies on top and/or to the sides of the urethral opening. Try lightly tickling the area with an index finger. If all goes well, a small bump may spring up: That's because the U-spot contains erectile tissue that is rising up to say, "Hey, thanks for that!"

ALL THUMBS

Fine with or without lubrication

Long before you delve deep into a woman's inner cathedral, you should spend plenty of time strolling around the outskirts, and this technique is a wonderful way to make the rounds. Resting your hands on her inner thighs, use the pads of your thumbs to caress the outer labia (the area to the sides of the vagina) from top to bottom with a motion like windshield wipers. Not only will this teasing touch get her temperature rising; the hand-to-thigh contact will help spread those sensations outward beyond the narrow confines of just the genitals for an even bigger buzz.

ON A ROLL

Best with lubrication

Using both hands, squeeze her outer labia between your thumbs and forefingers and roll the tissue in your hands. Essentially you're giving her outer labia a massage—and what area of the body *doesn't* enjoy a good rubdown? The results will be the same as if you were kneading any area of the body: You relax the tissue, improve circulation, and increase sensitivity.

THE ATOMIC CLOCK

Fine with or without lubrication

Like On a Roll, this technique massages around the vaginal opening but in a more targeted way that will help you suss out which area is the most rub-worthy. Envision a clock face on the vulva with twelve o'clock being right above the clitoris, three o'clock to one side of the outer labia, six o'clock below the vaginal opening, and so on. On every hour massage tiny circles (making sure you don't penetrate the vagina) and await her reaction at each stop. You may find that eight o'clock is her own personal witching hour, or that high noon gets her in party mode. Either way, once you have made the rounds, you'll have a much better understanding of what makes her tick and how to ring her bell.

TUG THE RUG

Fine with or without lubrication

These days pubic hair is often seen as nothing more than a hindrance—a curly jungle that obscures buried treasures, gets stuck in teeth, and all in all gives you a hard time. Still that bush does bring some unique perks in the turn-on department. Merely sift your fingers through her tresses, close your fingers around a good-sized patch, and pull. *Gently,* of course. Since hair follicles are rooted under the skin, you'll be stimulating nerve endings deep in her nether regions that your hands couldn't reach otherwise. That said, since this technique is *muy caliente,* treat it like a spice and use it sparingly.

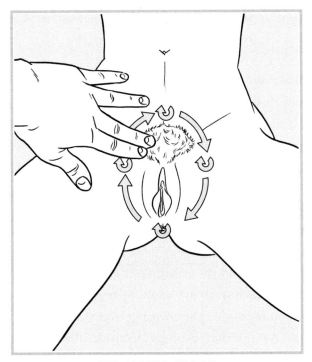

THE ATOMIC CLOCK

TEACHER'S PET

Best with lubrication

Given that the inner labia are the last things you pass on your way to the vagina, it makes sense that they're extremely sensitive, and that means she'll feel even the lightest caress here. Here's how to heat things up without slipping into overkill: Rest your hand on her mons pubis, with your fingers facing south and your middle finger resting between her inner labia. Curl your fingers toward your palm so that your middle finger caresses the inner labia from bottom to top. Meanwhile the heel of your palm should remain anchored to the mons; this will help control your movements and give your strokes a subtle quality that a free-roaming hand could never pull off.

THE SHIMMY

Must be done without lubrication

The inner labia may be sensitive, but they're also fairly elastic, and this quality can spark her tinderbox in an entirely new way. Using thumb and forefinger, pinch the inner labia together, gently stretch them taut, then wiggle them quickly from side to side. Not only will this send waves of sensation rippling through the area; it can also fire up another hot spot you might expect is too far off to be affected: the clitoris. That's because the inner labia don't just cover the vaginal opening; they extend all the way up to the crest of the vulva and are one with the clitoral hood. As a result, by tugging these two lips from side to side, you're causing the covering over the clitoris to shift back and forth and rub this nub just right. Consider it a sneaky way to put an orgasm imminently within your grasp. (Note: Not all women have inner labia long enough for you to grasp onto; if that's the case, try this technique with the outer labia.)

BY INVITATION ONLY

Best with lubrication

Of course, entering her vagina always feels fantastic. Rather than taking the initiative yourself to explore her inner corridors, turn the tables and let *her* take the lead. Firmly rest the flat of one fingertip on, but not in, the opening of the vagina. Then ask her to "invite" you in, which she can do by squeezing her pubococcygeal muscle, the same muscle she'd use to stop the flow of urine (if she's familiar with Kegel exercises, this is exactly the same thing). By squeezing these muscles she'll create a slight suction at the opening of the vagina that should draw you in. If her PC muscle isn't strong enough, she can also undulate her pelvis, thus using your finger to penetrate herself (this is where belly dancing lessons might come in handy). No matter how she does it, this process turns *her* into the aggressor in the penetration process, a role reversal that you may both find arousing.

THE WINDUP

Best with lubrication

Once inside the vagina, many people treat their hand like a penis, moving in and out in a thrusting motion. We're not saying this isn't nice, but after years or decades of this technique, she's dying, *dying,* for something new. So instead insert a finger (or two if she wishes) and slowly rotate your wrist—first clockwise, then counterclockwise, as far as it will turn. This will stimulate the vaginal walls laterally verses lengthwise, delivering a fresh sensation. For added variety, try twisting and thrusting at the same time, although you should be sure to start out slowly and see if she likes it.

VAGINA YOGA

Best with lubrication

Here's another technique we'll bet her vagina's never experienced, but that she will love once she feels the results. With one or two fingers fully inserted, slowly but firmly press on the back wall of the vaginal wall and hold for a count of five. Then take five to slowly press against the sides, then up against the front. This will stretch the vaginal tissue and provide a uniquely pleasurable sensation—and, of course, prep the area for a whole lot more in the penetration department, which we're sure you'll be glad to fulfill.

ROCK THE CASBAH

Best with lubrication

Create a C with your thumb and index finger. Insert your index finger into her vagina and rest your thumb on the clitoris so that the crook is nestled between the inner labia. Then start rocking your wrist from side to side. This should stimulate all three areas—clitoris, inner labia, and vagina.

RAISE THE ROOF

Best with lubrication

This technique allows you to jump-start her G-spot—that infamous erogenous zone inside the vaginal canal that can trigger intense sensations and may even cause women to ejaculate. In spite of its phenomenal reputation, the G-spot continues to remain a mystery for many couples. While we can attribute some of the cluelessness to the fact that not all women are equally sensitive here, many partners may merely be looking in the wrong place or not offering the right kind of stimulation. Allow us to shed some light on the operation of the G-spot.

First off, as a reminder, make sure she has hit the john. G-spot stimulation can feel strikingly similar to the urge to urinate, so by peeing beforehand she can relax knowing that whatever she feels going forward is G-spot-related rather than pee-related. While she's lying on her back, insert your index or middle finger (or both if she wishes) into the vagina. With your palm facing up, curl your finger(s) up against the roof of the vagina, feeling for a rough, quarter-sized patch anywhere from one to three inches in. Once you find it, exert pressure here by crooking your finger in a come-hither motion. At first she may feel nothing special or the movement might feel a little uncomfortable, but be patient and make sure she keeps breathing deeply. After a few minutes she may feel a tickle or the urge to urinate (which she'll know is false). Keep at it and you may soon be rewarded with the aforementioned splashy finale—and remember, female ejaculate is not urine, so don't worry if it gets on the sheets or elsewhere.

RAISE THE ROOF II

Best with lubrication

If you have discovered her G-spot and enjoyed the results, try delving deeper in search of the anterior fornix erogenous zone, or A-spot. This spongy area on the front wall of her vagina will feel similar to the G-spot, but it is located three to four inches in (to reach it, you're best off using your middle finger since it's the longest). As with the original Raise the Roof technique, ask her to lie on her back then insert your finger palm up, feeling against the roof of the vagina. Once you encounter a rough patch three to four inches in, crook your finger in a come-hither motion.

Arousing the A-spot can also cause women to ejaculate, although keep in mind that sensitivity levels vary. If you find that neither her G-spot nor her A-spot bring on the waterworks you were hoping for, consider stimulating these areas in conjunction with one of her more reliable hot spots, such as her clitoris.

SAND THE FLOOR

Best with lubrication

While many of the techniques we teach focus on the roof of the vagina since that's where so many hot spots reside, the bottom (or back wall) of the vagina is nothing to scoff at, either. That's because right behind it lies the anal canal—another supersensitive area that we'll deal with more directly in chapter 9. Meanwhile, though, you might be interested to know that you can *in*directly stimulate her back alley with this maneuver.

Have your partner lie faceup and slowly insert your index or middle finger into the vagina with your palm facing down. Press down on the floor of the vagina, massaging in small circles. In addition to perking up her fanny-side corridor, we've found that this technique can cause women to produce more natural lubrication, perhaps due to secretions from the nearby Skenes gland. Just keep in mind the intensity of response varies from person to person. In some women nothing will happen; others will melt with pleasure.

TRIPLE TREAT
Best with lubrication

This technique takes coordination, but it's well worth the effort, since it hits not just one or two but *three* erogenous zones at once: the G-spot, the A-spot, and the C-spot (aka her clitoris). To accomplish this feat of manual dexterity, start by slowly inserting your index and middle fingers into the vagina at the same time (but only if she finds two fingers comfortable and is warmed up enough to enjoy it). Place your index finger on the G-spot and your middle finger on the A-spot, then crook both fingers in a come-hither motion. Meanwhile place the thumb of that same hand on the clitoris and massage in small circles. Just think: Given that you're hitting three times as many nerve endings as you would if you'd honed in on one moan-worthy zone alone, you have single-handedly tripled your chances of sending her pleasure skyward.

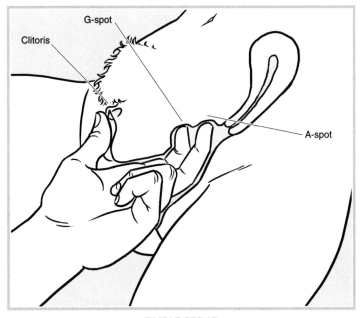

TRIPLE TREAT

CLITORIS SANDWICH

Best with lubrication

The G-spot and A-spot aren't the only bundles of nerves lying along the front wall of the vaginal canal. Press upward hard enough and you can also stimulate the root of the clitoris—which, you may recall, extends three to four inches into the pelvic cavity. To hit this hard-to-reach spot, you'll need both hands in on the action: one on top handling the visible portion of the clitoris, and one on the bottom stimulating the base of the clitoris from inside the vagina, sandwiching the clitoris from both sides. On top, squeeze the clitoral shaft between the pads or knuckles of your index and middle fingers.

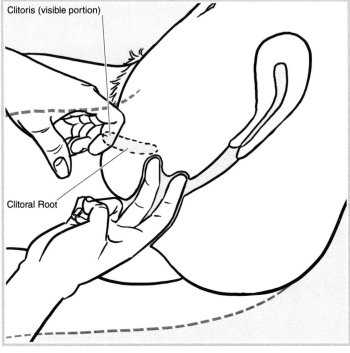

Clitoris (visible portion)

Clitoral Root

CLITORIS SANDWICH

Then, if you can, move your hand up and down as if you were stroking along the shaft. Meanwhile insert two fingers into the vaginal canal with your palm facing up, spread your fingers in a V, and press up against the front wall in a come-hither motion. Try to bring both hands closer together, and you should have the clitoral root sandwiched neatly between them.

FISTING: HOW TO MAKE IT FEEL PHENOMENAL

Fisting—where you insert your entire hand inside the vagina—may sound painful or all but impossible to perform on the woman you're with. And yet if your partner wants to give it a go and you take the right steps, it can be an intensely pleasurable experience. If you and your partner are curious, follow these pointers to ensure things go smoothly.

USE LOTS OF LUBE—With fisting, lubricant is downright essential, since it cuts down on friction and gives your fingers easier entry. That said, you should not use lube as an excuse to push past her comfort zone. Throughout the process take it slow and stay in close communication with your partner about what feels good. If at any point she indicates she's uncomfortable, stop immediately. Our motto is no pain, no pain.

FIRST STEP: STRETCH—Obviously your whole hand can't just head on in and expect a warm welcome. Instead start with one finger as usual and prep the area by stretching it. Press your finger against the vaginal wall—top, sides, and bottom—holding each stretch for at least five seconds. If this relaxes the area enough that you can easily insert two fingers (your second and third are ideal), repeat the same stretch on the vaginal walls. If you find you can't easily insert two fingers, don't force it. Either repeat the first step again or move on to other activities.

MAKE SURE SHE BREATHES DEEPLY—Deep breathing will help relax the vaginal muscles, thereby increasing their flexibility. Ask her to slowly inhale and exhale as you perform each stretch and with luck you should feel the tissue slowly expand.

STIMULATE WHILE YOU STRETCH—Don't get so caught up in the penetration process that you forget to turn her on in other ways. Be sure to stroke or lick some of her other hot spots—clitoris, breasts, nipples—while you gradually work your way in. Arouse her and this will increase blood flow to the pelvic area, making the tissue here even more pliable.

SLOWLY ADD FINGERS FOLLOWING HER LEAD—If your partner's vagina relaxes enough that it appears there's room for more than two fingers, it's time to get your thumb in on the action. Press the pad of your thumb between your middle and third fingers so your hand looks like a duck. Then slowly insert these three fingers into the vagina and resume stretching as usual. If all goes well proceed to inserting your index, middle, and fourth finger, then those three fingers with the thumb, then adding the pinky at the end. Make sure you're stretching, and she's breathing, and that you're not pushing past what she finds pleasurable.

YOU'RE IN! NOW WHAT?—Once all five fingers are inside the vagina, you may be wondering what's next. The funny thing is, *nothing* really needs to happen. Just keep your hand stationary and hang out for a while. More advanced fisters might consider moving their wrist in tiny circles, but keep in mind that your goal isn't to rub the vagina as you usually do—the fact that you're stretching the tissue may feel incredible enough. Combine that with a few licks or caresses on some of her other hot spots. All too soon you may start feeling her vaginal muscles contract around your hand as she reaches her peak.

MAKE A GRACEFUL EXIT—Once your partner's had her fill, you'll want to withdraw *very* slowly. Do not pull out—instead, let her push you out. Keeping your hand relaxed, ask her to inhale deeply and contract her PC muscle and then bear down as she exhales. Bit by bit, this should expel your hand from her vagina.

EXPLORE THE BACK DOOR

A GUIDE TO ANAL PLEASURES

The most important thing, the single most important thing when you're talking about wanting to progress forward with any kind of anal erotic play is desire. You must, must do this because you want to do it . . . Of all the parts of your body, nothing knows a liar like your anus. So if your mind is saying "Yes! Yes!" and your heart is saying "No! No!" your anus will always listen to your heart. —NINA HARTLEY

Some of you may have skipped straight to this chapter because you know this is gonna be good. Others may be wincing and thinking of flipping the page but are still reading because deep, deep down, you're thinking the exact same thing: *Hmm, maybe this is gonna be good.* Either way, you've come to the right place.

Let's start with the facts: The anus contains more nerve endings than any other area of the body except for the genitals. That means that its capacity to feel pleasure is astronomical, and this holds true whether you're man or woman, gay or straight, bisexual, transsexual, pansexual, or somewhere in between—an anus is an anus is an anus. Venture into this wild, wonderful frontier, and a host of moan-making, bed-quaking sensations await. And as always, your hands play a crucial role in making that happen.

Whether you are a back door virgin or an anal aficionado looking for new ideas, this chapter will leave everyone satisfied (in fact, anal massage can relax the entire body). Even if your partner is adamant that nothing enter the exit, we've provided plenty of techniques you can try *around* the aperture that will feel amazing even if you never head in. Anal play may not be for everyone, but honestly, how do you know one way or the other until you learn the right steps and give it a try? If you and your partner agree, let's get this party started.

PREPPING FOR THE PLUNGE: TIPS TO ENSURE PAINLESS PLAY

Anal play is kind of like skydiving: Follow protocol and the experience can be exhilarating. Flout the rules and you will most likely crash and burn. If you want to avoid becoming a cautionary tale that feeds the back door's bad rap, you've got to take a few safeguards seriously. Heed this advice to up the odds you'll have a rave-worthy trip.

Go Slow

We're talking snail's-pace slow. The anus is not to be entered with abandon—in fact, on most people (especially the uninitiated) it might be best if it is not entered at all, at least at first. Instead stick to frolicking on the outskirts, which are also sensitive and will enjoy the attention. Once you do circle in toward the anal star, *do not barge in.* The anus should *let* you in, or else you have no business being in there at all. Throughout the process, make sure your partner is breathing deep, since this will help relax the back channel.

Use Lube—Lots of It

The anus isn't naturally lubricated, so it's BYOL (Bring Your Own Lube). This will help you ease into your entry without making your partner uncomfortable (although you shouldn't use lube as an excuse to shoehorn in; listen to your partner's body and proceed at his or her pace). To protect against STDs, wear a condom, dental dam, or latex glove over your finger (for more details on lube and protective coverings, turn to chapter 2).

Get Anal About Your Anatomy

If you've never been up the hindquarters, it can help if you know what to expect along the way. Here's a rundown of the coming attractions in order of appearance.

The Outer Sphincter: Your first stop, of course, is the outer sphincter muscle—that cute little pucker between your partner's butt cheeks. Since this ringlike muscle is controlled by the central nervous system, people can voluntarily tighten or relax this orifice on command (although it may take practice).

The Inner Sphincter: Insert your finger past sphincter 1, and about one to two centimeters in you'll encounter another sphincter. Unlike the first, this sphincter is controlled by the autonomic nervous system, which means the person it belongs to can't really will it to do what he or she wants—and neither can you. So how do you edge past? Just

WORRIED ABOUT THE CRAP FACTOR? HOW TO DEAL

He's, like, trying to sell me on [anal sex] being "natural." I'm like, "Um, first of all, doody comes out of there, okay? And second of all, fucking doody comes out of there." I don't need two reasons when doody's involved.

—SARAH SILVERMAN

There's no getting around the fact that the anus is, well, an anus with all that entails. But provided you prep right, nine times out of ten you'll find nary a trace of excrement. Your first preventative measure has to do with your diet: If you have a hunch you'll delve into anal territory in the next day or two, eating fiber will help keep your highway debris-free (some natural sources of fiber include fresh fruits and vegetables, raw spinach, whole grains, legumes, and nuts, or ask for suggestions at your local health food store).

For further flawlessness, hop in the shower and wash where the sun don't shine. That's right, insert a finger in your bum as far as is comfortable to clear the area (don't forget to trim your fingernails first and be sure to rinse thoroughly since sudsy residue can be irritating and can disturb the bacterial balance in the rectum). Exploring your own alleyway has an added benefit: You'll know what to expect—both as the penetrator and the penetratee—and that's priceless.

Still, remember that no matter how much you scrub and plan ahead, sometimes shit happens. Keeping baby wipes handy can help with minor touch-ups during the action.

camp out at its doorstep. Lightly press on the sphincter and wait for an opening. Eventually it should let you in.

The Rectum: Beyond these two ring-shaped gatekeepers lies the rectum—a relatively roomier corridor ranging in length from four to six inches. More S-shaped than straight, the rectum is filled with some pretty sensitive spots. On men there's the prostate gland around three inches in; on women you can jump-start the G-spot, which lies right next door in the vaginal canal. Another thing you'll be glad to know about the rectum is that poop doesn't park here. In general, feces are stored further up in the colon, and the rectum is probably as far as your fingers will be able (or want) to go.

Watch Out for Infections

Even squeaky-clean anuses can contain harmful bacteria. As a result, nothing that has been up the back chute—finger, penis, sex toy, or whatever—should subsequently enter the vagina, since the bacteria from the anus can cause an infection. To avoid trouble, make a point of using one hand exclusively in the front slot and your other hand out back, or put a condom over your finger or use a vinyl glove and remove it once you're done with fanny fun. You'll also want to keep lube from spreading from the anus to the vagina (especially if she's lying on her stomach); placing a small hand towel between her legs works well as added protection.

Attention Straight Couples:
Anal Play Does Not Mean He's Gay

While back road excursions have gained popularity among straight couples, the prospect can still spark some anxiety. If a man really, *really* likes it, does that mean he's secretly batting for his own team? We're not gender psychologists, but we think that's highly unlikely. Your hands are powerful, but not *that* powerful. Anal penetration may feel good, but straight (and bi) men are attracted to women for a whole slew of reasons—a finger up his butt isn't going to change that. In fact, ladies, given it's *your* finger, this will merely give him one more reason to worship the ground *you* walk on. So stop worrying and just thank your stars he's having the time of his life.

TRICKS THAT'LL TICKLE THAT TUSH

The following techniques fall into two camps. The first group of maneuvers loiters *around* the back door but doesn't enter. This can be a pleasurable sensation in its own right, and a great way to test the waters and warm up for more in-depth work. After that, we've included some techniques that take you a little deeper. All techniques are fine to try on both men and women except where indicated otherwise. Just remember, as Margaret Cho once said, "Everyone's anus is a little bit different. They're like snowflakes." So check in with your partner frequently to make sure you're rubbing that rear the right way.

Non-penetrative Techniques

ANAL YOGA
Fine with or without lubrication
Slowly spread the butt cheeks with both hands and place your thumbs on each side of the anus. Pressing down gently, pull your thumbs gradually apart. Ask your partner to inhale deeply, then exhale, at which point your thumbs should return back to their starting position. Then do the exact same thing again—the breathing, the stretching—but inch your thumbs to more of a diagonal position around the anus and pull diagonally, then inch your thumbs right above and below the anus and pull up and down. Remember, your

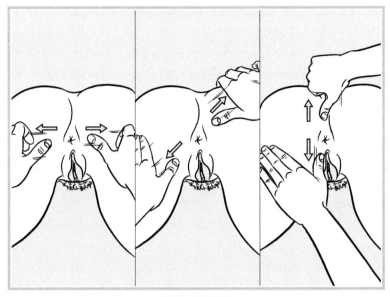

ANAL YOGA

partner's breathing is key; without it his or her anus might not relax at all. Take your time and this technique will stretch and stimulate the area, which can serve as the perfect opening act, so to speak.

BACK DOOR FOR BEGINNERS
Fine with or without lubrication

For people who aren't used to anyone *touching* their anus, much less entering it, it's crucial you get them accustomed to the sensation before diving in. Here's how: Merely rest your hand between the butt cheeks so the tip of your middle finger is touching the anus. Rest your other hand on the sacrum—the bone just above the butt crack that, when touched, can get energy flowing throughout the pelvic region, which is bound to work in your favor. Keeping both hands still, ask your partner to breathe deep and imagine he or she is inhaling and exhaling through the anus. Sure it sounds weird, but it can help release tons of tension that is often stored here and can help open all kinds of doors. This technique is also a great way to end a session of anal penetration, since rather than brusquely beating a fast retreat, you can stay connected and ease out of this intimate encounter.

POSTERIOR IN PRAYER
Lots of lubrication a must

Put your hands together as if you were praying and place them in the crack between your partner's butt cheeks. Then move them back and forth along this crease in a slow sawing motion (if you're doing this on a woman, saw only in an upward motion to avoid getting lubrication from the anus into the vagina). Since you're rubbing the entryway but not intruding, this technique is also a pleasurable preliminary move.

SWIMMING UPSTREAM
Lots of lubrication a must

This technique is similar to Posterior in Prayer, only you undulate your hands as if they were a salmon wiggling its way up a river. This will set off a cascade of nerve endings along the butt's banks.

TWIDDLING YOUR THUMBS
Best with lubrication

Try twiddling your thumbs on the anus one right after the other. Start slow—say, each thumb pad contacting the anus once per second—and if your partner's enjoying it, slowly build up speed (thumb-twiddling masters might be able to get their thumb pads on the anus up to three times per second). Consider it the equivalent of knocking: It may earn you an invitation on in.

Penetrative Techniques

ACCESS GRANTED
Lots of lubrication a must
Once you've tried the non-penetrative anal techniques and your partner has signaled in so many words, signs, or moans that he or she is ready for more, it may be time to head in. Here's how: Rest one finger on the anus and very gently apply pressure, allowing your partner to draw you in. *Do not push in*—allow the anus to *let* you in. Once the tip of your finger has made it past the external anal sphincter, hold still for at least thirty seconds so your partner can get used to the sensation. Even without movement, penetration alone will feel pleasurable, and you don't want to rush the process. The slower your pace, the more you can both relish the experience.

ROUND TWO
Lots of lubrication a must
Once you're past the first sphincter, it's time to contend with sphincter 2, which should lie one to two centimeters farther inside on most people. As with the first sphincter, never force entry. Just hang out there, with your finger lightly pressing against the opening. Even this simple holding pattern will feel phenomenal. After a while, sphincter 2 may mellow and allow you a little deeper.

ROCK AROUND THE ANUS

Lots of lubrication a must

Once you've made it past both sphincters, you may notice that things open up a little—and it's time to start exploring. Envisioning a clock face along the rectum's outer edges, press along each hour. Try massaging small circles at each stop, closely gauging your partner's reaction. If you two are up for talking, even better. Describe what you're doing ("I'm pressing/rubbing at eight o'clock") and ask how it feels. This will help you pinpoint exactly which spots carry the highest sexual charge.

THE PROSTATE TICKLER (FOR MEN ONLY)

Lots of lubrication a must

On men, one special area of interest in the anus is the prostate—a highly sensitive gland located along the front wall around three inches in. If your partner is lying facedown, you can find the prostate by pressing down toward the floor; it should feel like a walnut-sized bump (keep in mind that the prostate can swell and become easier to locate once a guy is already aroused, so if you're having trouble finding it, consider working on other areas of his anatomy then checking back later). Once you've located the prostate, you can stimulate it by crooking your finger in a come-hither motion. Prepare to make him googly-eyed with pleasure; some men can reach orgasm through stimulation of the prostate alone.

HUGGING THE PROSTATE (FOR MEN ONLY)

Lots of lubrication a must

While massaging the prostate gland through the anus feels amazing, there's a way to double his pleasure, and here's the secret. Remember how the prostate can also be stimulated by pressing up on the perineum, the patch of flesh between his testicles and anus? Do that

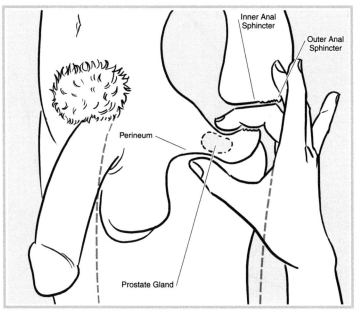

HUGGING THE PROSTATE

while penetrating him anally, and you can stimulate this extra-sensitive gland from *both* sides. To do it, create a C with your thumb and middle finger. Insert your middle finger into the anus and press down on the prostate while pressing up on the perineum with your thumb. Move your whole hand in small circles, and you'll have one puddle of satisfied man on your hands in no time.

JAZZING THE G-SPOT (FOR WOMEN ONLY)

Lots of lubrication a must

While women will find anal penetration pleasurable purely because the opening is loaded with nerve endings, there's another secret trigger point buried deeper within: the G-spot.

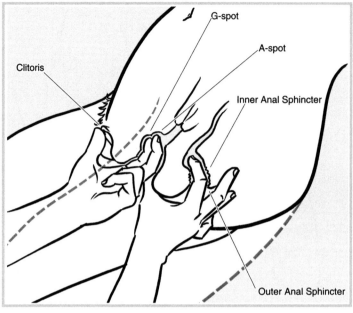

QUADRUPLE DELIGHT

That's right, this well-known erogenous zone is accessible through the rectum as well as the vagina. To reach it, have her lie on her stomach while you insert a finger into the anus palm down. Once you're around three inches in, press down toward the floor and crook your finger in a come-hither motion. In our classes we've seen women achieve orgasm this way, so consider making a special trip to check it out.

THE QUADRUPLE DELIGHT (FOR WOMEN ONLY)

Lots of lubrication a must

To start, make sure she's lying faceup, ideally with her legs raised so the backs of her knees or her feet are resting on your chest or shoulders. Insert a well-lubed finger into her anus, making sure she's warmed up before you delve deep. Then with your other hand insert your middle and index fingers in her vagina so they're touching the G-spot and A-spot. Finally, place the thumb of that same hand on the clitoris. Then start moving all fingers involved in small circles or however she likes it best. In effect, you're hitting *four* erogenous zones at once. And that's bound to be a grand slam arousal-wise.

PUTTING IT ALL TOGETHER

HOW YOUR HANDS CAN MAKE INTERCOURSE, ORAL SEX, AND EVERY IN-BED ACTIVITY HOTTER THAN EVER

Love is the answer, but while you are waiting for the answer, sex raises some pretty good questions. —WOODY ALLEN

Congratulations—if you've been reading up until this point, you now know more than a *hundred ways* to handle every hot spot on the body with mind-blowing results. But let's not stop there. One of the best things about your hands is that they play well with others and can be easily incorporated into all areas of your sex life, from intercourse to oral sex and beyond. In fact, pretty much *anything* you could imagine doing in bed can be made much hotter if your mitts are in the picture. So it's time to start getting fancy.

As you read on, you'll quickly notice that these all-in-one extravaganzas are built on the manual moves you learned in chapters 4, 6, 8, and 9 (so if you find yourself needing more guidance on how to do these techniques, feel free to flip back to those chapters for a refresher).

At first, the coordination involved in some of these combinations may be a bit challenging, kind of like patting your head and rubbing your stomach at the same time. But after a few tries you should be able to get the hang of it. Keep in mind, this list is by no means a *complete* inventory of all the amazing things your hands can do during a close encounter, and that good communication and connection matter way more than any trick you might have up your sleeve. So consider these ideas a launching pad for your new, improved sex life from which you can explore and experiment further—you'll find your hands will become virtuosos at improvising from here on out. So if you and your partner feel ready to embark on some of the wildest rides of your life, read on, fasten your seatbelts, and have fun.

HANDS + MOUTH = AMAZING ORAL SEX

Let's do the math: Your mouth is capable of delivering a wild, wet wonderland of sensations. Mix that in with the many skills your hands now possess and the pleasure possibilities are virtually infinite. Even if you usually use your hands during oral sex to a certain extent, chances are you've barely scratched the surface of all the amazing ways your hands and kisser can work in tandem. It's time to open your eyes to all of your options. To kick things off, let's fill you in on a few general principles to keep in mind whenever you head downtown.

Your Hands Can Arouse What Your Mouth Can't Reach
Your mouth is fairly small compared to the genitals, which means that whatever it's licking, sucking, or nibbling, a lot of randy real estate gets left high and dry (if you've ever tried taking an entire penis in your mouth or tried reaching a woman's G-spot with your tongue,

we think you know what we mean). Get your hands to help out, though, and problem solved: If your tongue is on clitoris duty, your fingers can provide some pleasurable penetration down below; or if your mouth can only manage to take in the first third of the penis, wrap your hands around the rest. And since your hands are pros at mimicking how your mouth and tongue feel, your recipient will enjoy both sensations equally and will merely be amazed at just how much territory you're turning on.

Your Hands Can Free Up Your Kisser to Try New Things

If your mouth goes it alone and is the sole source of stimulation, it may feel a lot of pressure to stick with the old standbys (licking her clitoris, sucking his shaft) since these moves are almost guaranteed to satisfy. Let your hands step in and take over these essential stimulation duties, however, and your lips and tongue can start getting creative. Since the basics are covered, they can start experimenting with what one would typically consider add-on features such as cute little tongue swipes on his testicles or some playful pressure on her perineum. The result: a much more eclectic oral sex experience that is bound to leave your recipient satisfied.

Your Hands Can Teach Your Mouth a Thing or Two

Your lips and tongue may already know some pretty cool moves, but have you exhausted *all* of the possibilities? To expand your horizons, turn to your hands for pointers. Flip through chapters 6 and 8 and try giving your mouth a crack at a manual move. On women, try Ringing the Doorbell (point your tongue and press down on the clitoris) or The Shimmy (take the inner labia in your mouth—a bit of suction can help—and wiggle your head from side to side). On men, try Rattle On (open your mouth wide and bounce the head of the penis around inside, just be careful of your teeth) or Scrotum Yoga (gently pinch the middle seam of the scrotum between your lips and pull). By letting your mouth follow in your hands' footsteps, you can begin thinking outside the box of your typical oral sex maneuvers and open doors to an array of new sensations.

Your Hands Can Fill In While Your Mouth Takes Breaks

If your tongue tires of wiggling, your lips start quivering, or your neck gets a crick, yet again, this is an instance where your hands can come to the rescue. Let your hands take over for a while so your mouth can rest up. And again, since your hands and mouth deliver strikingly similar sensations, your partner won't care whether you're using one or the other. He or she will just be glad you can keep going . . . and going . . . and going!

Your Recipient Can Lend a Hand, Too

Sometimes it's nice to let your partner kick back and not lift a finger while you dine out down below. It's also fine if your partner wants to pitch in and make this more of a mutual pleasure fest. He or she can give you a scalp massage, shoulder rub, or (if your position makes it possible) reach down and start petting your genitals. Finally, if they're so inclined, oral sex recipients can put their hands on themselves. A man can play with his testicles while you fool around with his penis; a woman can massage her breasts or clitoris while you're off on a quest for her G-spot. Since some people might feel strange or self-conscious touching themselves during sex, you may want to reassure your partner by saying what a turn-on it would be to see such a sexy sight. Honestly, as long as the end result is oodles of pleasure, who cares whose hands are responsible? Our opinion is, the more hands, the merrier!

You Should *Still* Use Lube

Just because your mouth is on the scene doesn't mean it should have to provide all the slip 'n' slide for a satisfying experience. And besides, saliva evaporates quickly, so you're bound to run dry before you've finished the job. If the taste of lube isn't to your liking, try coconut oil (which has antifungal properties and reportedly can keep the vaginal environment healthier) or a flavored brand of lube, such as the aptly named Good Head Gel (which comes in mint or cherry) or Sliquid Swirl (available in green apple, blue raspberry, or cherry vanilla). Just keep in mind that some women's vaginal environments may have a bad reaction to sugar or other additives; if so, try a homeopathic alternative.

Experiment with Different Positions

Your partner may typically receive oral sex lying down on a bed with you hunched over his or her privates, but this position can become a pain in the neck—plus it limits your access to certain hot spots you might like hitting. Luckily, there are plenty of other ways to situate yourselves for a satisfying time downtown. Here are a few ideas:

- The recipient sitting on the edge of a chair or bed with legs spread, with you kneeling on the floor between them. Since this position allows you to keep your head and torso vertical, you can avoid straining your neck. If your partner scoots forward far enough, you've got better access to back areas, including the testicles, perineum, and (if the person raises his/her legs) the anus.

- The recipient standing, with you kneeling in front. This is also a non-neck-straining position; plus if your partner's legs are spread, this position provides better petting opportunities for the testicles, vagina, perineum, and/or anus.
- The recipient standing with one foot propped up on a chair or bed, and with you kneeling. Again, zero neck strain and access to all those nooks and crannies.
- You and the recipient lying on your sides in bed. Talk about relaxing—plus if you're up for a little 69 action where you swap oral sex at the same time, all of your hands will be free to roam.

ORAL SEX ON HIM: HAND-AND-MOUTH COMBOS HE'LL LOVE

If you thought your guy loved blow jobs already, wait'll he gets a load of the tricks you're about to learn now. If you've read chapter 6, you should already have a handle on the manual portion of these moves (feel free to refer back to that chapter when necessary); now all that's left is to add some mouth maneuvers. Here's how.

TICKLING THE FRENULUM

Best when he is erect, lubrication a must

Now that your hands can take over some stimulation duties, a prime place for them to start is the shaft. Using lube, wrap one or both hands around his pillar and start pumping. Meanwhile your mouth can turn to more detailed work, like licking the frenulum—an extra-sensitive erogenous zone located on the front side of the penis just below the head. Gently swipe your tongue from side to side on this tiny spot; for added variety use the underside of your tongue, which has a much silkier texture. When you combine this with your hands' actions, he may light up like a Christmas tree.

TAUT AS A DRUM

Best when he is erect, with or without lubrication

Begin this move just like The Juicer from chapter 6, where you hold his penis at the base and pull down. This will tug the skin taut, exposing more nerve endings and increasing his scepter's sensitivity. Now just about *any* move your mouth makes will feel even more scintillating. Try licking or sucking the head, and his heat-seeking missile will love every minute.

THE SOUND OF ONE PENIS CLAPPING

Fine when he is erect or soft, with or without lubrication

Stick out your tongue and flatten it. Then, keeping your head and tongue stationary, hold his penis at the base and quickly shake it from side to side so that the head slaps and slides against your tongue. This technique (a hybrid of Shake, Rattle, and Roll and Patty Cake from chapter 6) combines two very invigorating sensations: wild shaking, plus tiny tongue lashings. Together they'll send his nerve endings into a tizzy.

O MY

Best when he is erect, with lubrication

Curl your fingers into an O and place your lips around the edge. Then lower your hand and mouth onto his penis and move them up and down in unison. This classic move creates the illusion that you're taking *all* of him into your mouth when, in fact, your hand is doing most of the heavy lifting. If your mitts are well lubricated, this will only further convince him that your hands and mouth are one and the same.

SQUEEZE ME, TEASE ME

Best when he is erect, with or without lubrication

With your tongue circling the extra-sensitive head of the penis, take your thumb and forefinger and perform Cock Shiatsu from chapter 6: Form a ring around the base of the penis, tighten the ring for about one second, then release. Next, move your "ring" up half an inch and squeeze again, continuing up the shaft. Unlike your usual rubbing motion, this will stimulate tissue *underneath* the skin and boost circulation, leading to a bigger erection that will enjoy your teasing tongue licks up top all the more.

EVERY WHICH WAY BUT LOOSE

Best when he is erect, lubrication a must

This technique stimulates his penis in four directions—up, down, and side to side—which is sure to throw his lust meter for a loop. To do it, take the head of his penis in your mouth and move up and down while you take the shaft of his penis between your palms. Slide your hands side to side as if you were trying to start a fire or wrap one or both hands around the shaft and twist. Keep your hands and mouth in motion simultaneously, and it'll send him to an alternate pleasure plane.

THE PENIS WHISPERER

Best when he is erect, with or without lubrication

After doing any of the previously described maneuvers, grab his penis at the base and hold it still. Then pucker your lips and blow on the head. This will cause moisture to evaporate, which will give him chills. Consider it the perfect refreshing pick-me-up between rubdown rounds.

THE HUMMER

Fine when he is erect or soft, with or without lubrication

This technique combines Good Vibes from chapter 6 with a mouth move that will amplify its sexy effects. To start, place your fist against the area between his testicles and his anus. Start vibrating your fist, which will stimulate his perineum and the prostate gland underneath. At the same time take his penis in your mouth and start humming (or moaning if that feels more natural). Your vibrating vocal chords will transmit pleasurable ripples throughout his package. These vibrations paired with the pulses reverberating up from his perineum are bound to give him a buzz. If he moans on top of it, all the better.

TESTICLE TEASER

Best when he is erect, with or without lubrication

Using your thumb and index finger, form a ring around the base of the testicles and gently pull them away from his body so that the skin is taut. This exposes more nerve endings, upping the area's sensitivity levels. Start licking his family jewels and you'll have one grateful guy on your hands.

ON THE EDGE

Best when he is erect, with or without lubrication

Similar to the Testicle Teaser, this move also requires that you encircle the base of his scrotum and gently pull it away from his body. Only this time you've got an entirely different purpose in mind: to delay ejaculation. Since these two little sperm factories tend to ride up right before he goes off the deep end, gently pulling them away from the body will help keep his grand finale on hold. Take his penis in your mouth and see how long you can keep him in this delicious limbo—the longer, the better.

LORD OF THE RINGS

Best when he is erect, with or without lubrication

This move is a combination of the Testicle Teaser and Taut as a Drum. With one hand, form a ring around the base of the penis and slowly pull down; with your other hand form a ring around the base of his testicles and gently tug them away from his body. Now that the skin in both areas is stretched taut and primed for pleasure, let your tongue flit back and forth between them.

MORE PROSTATE, PLEASE

Fine when he is erect or soft, lots of lubrication a must

This technique combines oral sex with some rear end activity, so make sure you've read chapter 9 before trying it. Out back, slowly insert a finger into the anus and perform The Prostate Tickler, where you crook your finger in a come-hither motion on the front wall of the rectum around three inches in. Meanwhile, stimulate the prostate from the *outside* as well by pressing up on the perineum, the area between his anus and his testicles. Finally, let your mouth work its magic up front by taking the head of his penis in your mouth.

ORAL SEX ON HER: HAND-AND-MOUTH COMBOS SHE'LL LOVE

Treating a woman to an otherworldly oral sex experience is a cinch when your hands are involved. In chapter 8 we showed you all the amazing things your palms and fingers can do down below (for a refresher turn back to that chapter). In this section we'll show you how to weave in some mouth maneuvers. Together they may feel so good she may start racking up orgasms galore.

PULLING DOWN THE HOOD

Fine with or without lubrication

Many times a mouth's ability to send a woman to cosmic heights goes untapped purely because one of her most sensitive spots—the clitoris—remains hidden under the clitoral hood. The solution: Use one or both hands to push up on the mons pubis, the fleshy mound up top that is covered in pubic hair. This will cause the clitoral hood to withdraw, exposing the pink kernel of her clit to whatever your mouth has in mind. Start with light licks, and if that goes well let your tongue take a crack at a few manual moves, such as gently running the flat of your tongue across the head of the clitoris. Just keep in mind that when the clitoris is exposed like this it's *extremely* sensitive. Treat it with the utmost care and check in with your partner constantly.

LITTLE EARTHQUAKE WITH LICKS

Fine with or without lubrication

Rest the heel of your palm on her lower stomach so that your curled fingers rest on her mons pubis. Then drum your fingers on top of the mons. At the same time, start licking the clitoris, letting your tongue flicker quickly over her love nub. Together these two techniques will send pleasurable tremors throughout the area.

LITTLE EARTHQUAKE TIMES TWO

Fine with or without lubrication

This technique is just like Little Earthquake with Licks, where you drum your fingers on top of her mons. Only instead of licking the clitoris, place your lips around this little nub and start humming or moaning. The vibration from your vocal cords will feel amazing (similar to the effects of a battery-powered sex toy), and your finger drumming above will only amplify those effects.

BIG EARTHQUAKE WITH BENEFITS
Fine with or without lubrication

Place the tip of your tongue on the clitoris and hold it stationary. Meanwhile, cup the mons pubis in one hand and press down and jiggle the mons from side to side. Keep your hand relaxed to ensure bigger vibrations. Not only will the jiggling feel amazing by itself, but since you're moving the vulva and clit against the tongue, you're essentially licking this supersensitive button without having to wiggle your tongue one inch. How's that for making your mouth's job easy?

G-SPOT/C-SPOT COMBO
Best with lubrication

Given that all of the previous turn-on techniques require just one of your hands, that means your other hand is still free, and we know exactly where it should go. Send it in search of her G-spot—an erogenous zone on the front wall of her vagina—by inserting a finger and exploring inside for a rough quarter-sized patch one to three inches in. Once you find it, crook your finger in a come-hither motion (for more details turn to chapter 8 and see Raise the Roof). Meanwhile use your other hand and your mouth to stimulate the clitoris via any of the aforementioned moves.

SKINNY DIPPING
Best without lubrication

Vulva Yoga—a technique from chapter 8 where you gently grasp the outer labia between thumb and fingers and pull down toward her feet—is a veritable boon as far as oral sex is concerned. Not only does this technique stretch and stimulate the outer environs; it also gives your tongue incredible access to the extra-sensitive area in between, where the inner labia and clitoris are located. To give it a try, pinch the outer labia, pull slowly, then run your tongue along the interior.

TUG THE RUG II

Best without lubrication

This technique is similar to Skinny Dipping, but instead of targeting the outer labia, gently grab the pubic hair on each side (the bigger the chunk, the better) and *very* gradually pull toward her feet. As with the previous technique, this will also expose the vulva's inner environs to your tongue tricks—and the hair tug adds an extra shot of va-va-voom.

DO I TURN U ON?

Fine with or without lubrication

The U-spot—an erogenous zone located on top and to the sides of the urethral opening—would probably love a little tongue action. To deliver, spread the inner labia with your fingers and scan the area for a tiny hole. That's the urethra, which means you've found the U-spot, too. Keeping the inner labia open, flick your tongue across the area. To mix things up, try using the underside of your tongue, which is silkier in texture than the rough upper side. It will feel U-nbelievable.

THE VAGINA WHISPERER

Fine with or without lubrication

Once you've aced any of the previously described moves and licked her into a frenzy, she'll go absolutely ballistic if you pull back and tease her a little. To switch gears, use two thumbs to lightly stroke her outer labia from top to bottom like windshield wipers. Meanwhile, with your mouth, blow on the area you were licking earlier. This stream of air will cause moisture to evaporate, resulting in a unique tingly sensation.

DOUBLE DELIGHT

Best with lubrication

Place a finger pad on but not in her vaginal opening and ask her to pull you in by contracting her pubococcygeal muscle, which can be located by stopping the flow of urine (for more details on this technique, turn to By Invitation Only in chapter 8). Meanwhile, take her clitoris in your mouth and start gently sucking on it. This will mean you're sucking on her while she's sucking on you, and that amounts to one intensely pleasurable exchange.

DOUBLE-DECKER CLITORIS SANDWICH DELUXE

Lots of lubrication a must

Similar to the Clitoris Sandwich in chapter 8, this technique stimulates the root of the clitoris, which lies three to four inches beneath the visible part of the clitoris, in the pelvic cavity. What's more, you may recall that this invisible lightning rod of nerve tissue can be reached from *within* the vagina as well as from the outside. Here's how to do both at once in a mouth-and-mitt combo that will likely light her up.

First, encircle the clitoris with your lips and gently suck on it so you've got a firm grip at its base. Meanwhile insert a finger or two into her vagina and press up against the front wall a few inches in. Then start wiggling your head *and* your fingers from side to side. Try to bring your mouth and your hand closer together, and you should have the clitoral root sandwiched neatly between them—which puts you in the position to serve up some very scrumptious sensations.

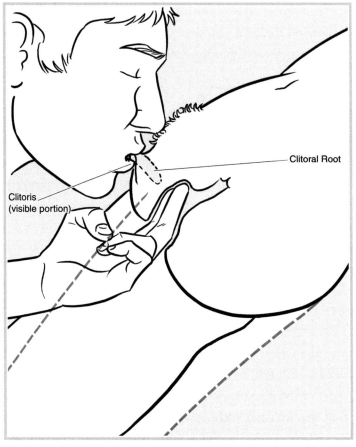

DOUBLE-DECKER CLITORIS SANDWICH DELUXE

UPSIDE-DOWN ORAL SEX

Fine with or without lubrication

Hands aren't only good at stroking, tickling, and tantalizing her hot spots. They're also great at holding and hoisting her body in ways that can make oral sex feel even *more* exhilarating. Case in point: Try lifting her butt off the bed and draping the backs of her legs over your

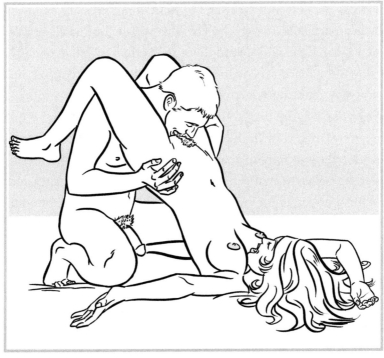

UPSIDE-DOWN ORAL SEX

shoulders so she's essentially lying at a steep angle with her head much lower than her feet. Then, let your tongue try some oral acrobatics (like, say, tracing circles around the clitoris with your tongue or lightly flicking your tongue over this supersensitive nub). Trust us, it's a stunner.

BOOTYLICIOUS

Lots of lubrication a must if anal penetration is included

If your gal enjoys having her tush played with, it's the perfect side dish if you're dining downtown. To warm her up, flatten your tongue as wide as possible and treat her to some long, slow ice cream licks from her perineum to her clitoris. Meanwhile, out back, squeeze a cheek in each hand and spread them apart, then together, one up and one down then vice versa. Once that has gotten her attention, up the intensity by pointing your tongue, inserting it into the vagina, and licking your way up between the inner labia to the clitoris, while in the rear you inch your middle fingers in toward the sides of the anus then stretch the skin here apart, then diagonally, then up and down. And if she's open to anal penetration, feel free to delve deeper and try crooking a finger along the front wall of the anal cavity around three inches in to stimulate her G-spot (for more details turn to chapter 9).

QUINTUPLE DELIGHT

Best with lubrication

Consider this move your manual tour de force, since it hits (count 'em) *five* supersensitive areas at once. With one hand, insert a well-lubed finger into the anus. With your other, insert your middle and index fingers into the vagina so they're touching the G-spot (located on the front wall one to three inches in) and the A-spot (also on the front wall three to four inches in). Place the thumb of that same hand on her U-spot (located on top of her urethral opening an inch or so above the vagina). Finally, put your tongue on clitoris duty. Start moving all appendages involved. What happens next will feel nothing short of transcendent.

INTERCOURSE: HOW YOUR HANDS CAN MAKE IT EXPLOSIVE

Granted, going hip to hip with someone you care about is a satisfying event unto itself. Get your hands in on the action, though, and you launch your pleasure potential to a new planet of possibilities. For starters, you may recall that two-thirds of women don't regularly reach orgasm through intercourse alone due to the fact that their clitoris doesn't receive sufficient stimulation (nor does her G-spot). That obstacle is easily overcome the minute you put your hands where she needs them most. And while men may think they couldn't be happier as long as they're humping away, your hands can up the ante for them too by providing even *more* sensory input. All in all, everyone benefits from a little manual action during the main attraction.

Before we get into specific techniques for making your mattress antics more mind-blowing, let's fill you in on a few general principles you should keep in mind no matter who's on top, bottom, or somewhere in between.

You Don't Have to Bump 'n' Grind the Whole Time

Couples often think that intercourse should be nonstop in-and-out thrusting. Not so. For one, that can be tiring. Two, being joined at the genitals is a sensation that can and should be savored in itself. And last but not least, certain manual moves are easier to do when your bodies aren't bobbing all over the place. If you think intercourse without thrusting sounds dull, remember, your hands will be offering plenty of stimulation to keep things plenty interesting.

You Can (Gasp!) Touch Yourself, Too, You Know

While people are generally raring to learn how to give their partner a hand during intercourse, they're often reluctant to use those newfound skills on themselves, perhaps because the thought of doing so makes them feel selfish or self-conscious. But our opinion is that unless your partner's a total monster, we doubt he or she is going to catch you caressing yourself and think it's weird or greedy. In fact, taking your pleasure into your own hands can be an incredible sight that your audience-of-one will appreciate. So why not put on a show?

Still, some people worry that touching themselves during sex conveys that their partner's in-bed abilities fall short of the mark—a silent accusation along the lines of *You can't get it right so I guess I should take care of matters myself.* But there are plenty of other reasons to handle your own hardware: Maybe it's just because your hands are better situated to push those particular buttons, or maybe you just want your partner to relax and enjoy the eye candy. Make your motive known and your partner won't feel sidelined and will be able to relish the fact that you're just very aroused right about now.

You Should Still Use Lube

Even with a vagina's naturally lubricating resources at your disposal, it may not be enough to slide all the way across the finish line. So please, since nothing hurts quite like too little lube and too much friction, keep a tube handy (for a rundown of some product options, turn to chapter 2).

Consider Reaching for Some Less Obvious Hot Spots

Genitals, breasts, butt—all are perfectly respectable places to put your hands when you do the deed. Still, they're hardly the only places that will appreciate some hands-on attention. The entire body is teaming with erogenous zones, and in chapter 4 we provided more than fifty techniques for turning them on. Tap into them and you will capitalize on the body's *full* potential for pleasure. That's why in our next section we'll show you how to use your hands *everywhere* during intercourse, not just below the belt. Our suggestions are just a sampling of all the places your hands can wander; feel free to expand from there.

ASSUME THE POSITION! HOW TO USE YOUR HANDS ON TOP, BOTTOM, AND EVERYWHERE IN BETWEEN

Given there are so many ways you can use your hands during intercourse, we've grouped our lessons according to the four most common sexual scenarios: the missionary position, woman on top, sex from behind, and sex side by side. For you adventurous folks who want to explore beyond that, we've included a fifth miscellaneous catchall category full of sexy surprises that'll make you blush. But first let's kick things off with the classic of classics—the missionary position—and provide some tips for how your hands can make it amazing.

Missionary Possible:
Manual Moves to Improve Man-on-Top Lovemaking

This position makes men feel like kings. That said, being top dog does come with a few challenges as far as your hands are concerned. Since the guy's arms are usually occupied propping up his torso so he doesn't crush his lovely bedfellow beneath, he is somewhat limited in how much his hands can do otherwise. That said, there are ways to work around this obstacle: Try a version of missionary where the man stands or kneels with his torso vertical, which eliminates his need for arm support. Or just leave the bulk of the handiwork to the bottom partner, whose hands are incredibly free to roam. Here are some techniques to try.

BARING THE SCEPTER

Most easily done from the bottom

Either partner can perform this technique, although the bottom person's hands may be able to pull it off more easily. Reaching down between your bodies, form a ring with thumb and forefinger around the base of the penis. Then pull down so the skin on the shaft is taut. This exposes more nerve endings and increases the penis's sensitivity (it can also help maintain his erection). Engage in intercourse with your hand still encircling the base. This technique is great at the outset of intercourse. Try it during those very first few thrusts and take it slow so he can savor every inch of the penetration process. It'll send his pleasure soaring.

UNCLOAKING THE CLIT

Most easily done from the bottom

Since a woman's clitoris is buried under the clitoral hood and cushiony mons pubis surrounding it, it's no wonder this tiny nub rarely receives enough stimulation during intercourse for a woman to arrive at the O station. Your hands, though, can help change that. Form a V with your index and middle finger, reach between your bodies, and press this V onto the mons pubis, with a finger to each side of the clitoris. Then pull up toward her belly, moving the skin with your hand. This should unveil the hard-to-reach clit in all its glory, exposing this little love button to a lot more action. You can easily keep your hand here throughout intercourse. If he starts speeding up thrusting as he approaches his peak, wiggle your wrist from side to side to give yourself a little extra in the stimulation department so that you can both reach your climactic peaks simultaneously.

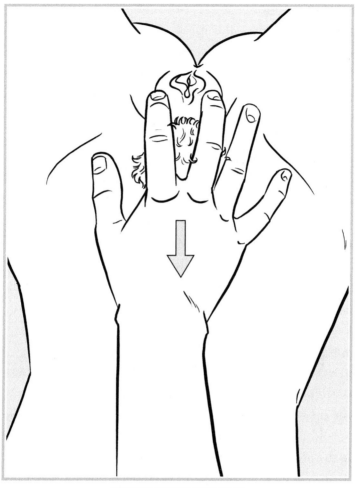

UNCLOAKING THE CLIT

CLOSING THE PEARLY GATES

Most easily done from the bottom

Extend both arms between your bodies and, using your fingertips, press the sides of the outer labia in toward the penis during intercourse. This provides a snugger fit—and more feel-good friction for both parties. To increase the effects, the bottom partner can close her legs together for an even tighter squeeze. Just remember, the tighter the aperture, the slower you should thrust to avoid overwhelming the nerve endings in the genital area.

POLISHING THE PEARLY GATES
Most easily done from the bottom

This technique is similar to Closing the Pearly Gates, where you press the outer labia in toward the penis, only with one very scintillating addition: To up the stimulation factor, massage the outer labia by moving your hands and the skin underneath in quarter-sized circles. His penis will feel the kneading as well. Slow down the pace of your lovemaking and you will be able to luxuriate in this move to the fullest.

SHAKE AND BAKE
Most easily done from the bottom

If you're craving a quick but stimulating break from intercourse, this move is the perfect titillating time-out. To do it the man withdraws and rests the tip of his penis on the clitoris. Then, reaching between your bodies, hold the base of the penis and shake it quickly from side to side so that the head hits the clit with every wiggle. In doing so, you'll be stimulating *both* heads at once—that of the clitoris and the penis.

JUMP-START THE SACRUM (HIM)
Must be done from the bottom

Reach around and place your hand on his sacrum—a triangular-shaped bone in the lower back that when stimulated can send signals via the sacral nerve straight into the genitals. To fire up this lust-inducing link, drum your fingertips on the area or press down on it with your entire palm. This will also get him penetrating you more deeply with every thrust. These two moves are probably easiest to do when the man is stationary for a few minutes taking a break. Try stimulating his sacrum while contracting your pubococcygeal or PC muscle (the one you use to stop urinating) and you may be surprised to find that's more than enough to keep him aroused.

PUSHING TUSH

Must be done from the bottom

If your guy enjoys having his back door explored, reach around with both hands and grab both cheeks. From there you can spread the cheeks apart, then together, one up one down then vice versa, or place your middle fingers to the sides of the anus then spread them apart, then diagonally, then up and down. If that gets him hankering for more, feel free to delve deeper; just make sure you've read the instructions in chapter 9 to ensure safe passage. During these moves (especially the more in-depth options), it's probably best that he remain still so your fingers can deftly perform their duties without too much jostling.

BUTTERING THE BOTTOM

Must be done from on top

To get set up for this move, the woman must raise her legs so that the man, who's kneeling below her butt, can prop his chest on the soles of her feet. Since she's now supporting his upper torso, his hands are free to start wandering—and this position presents the perfect body part for him to play with: her booty, which is now raised off the bed and easily within reach if he extends his arms under her legs. As with Pushing Tush, spreading the cheeks apart, then together, one up, one down then vice versa or placing your middle fingers to the sides of the anus and spreading them apart, diagonally, then up and down are great techniques to try. And if that leaves her wanting more, proceed to penetrative techniques. It's probably best to remain stationary so your hands out back can dazzle without too many distractions.

HAPPY SCISSORS
Must be done from on top

Heating up hot spots isn't your hands' only talent. They're also great at moving body parts where you want them, and this technique is a prime opportunity. During intercourse ask your partner to raise her legs, then hold an ankle in each hand. From there, you can spread her legs apart, hold them together, part them at 90 degrees—the options are endless. This move comes with a few benefits: One, your ankle hold gives you added traction, you can thrust much faster and deeper than usual (although you should take care that your partner is comfortable with the pace and pressure). Second, since the tendons of the legs pivot deep in the pelvic cavity, moving them around will subtly alter the below-the-belt sensations for you both.

FACE FORWARD
Must be done from on top

While a guy on top typically can't do much since his arms are occupied holding up his weight, by leaning on his elbows, he can free up his forearms for one *very* effective move. Looking into your partner's eyes, start massaging her face. Cheeks, temples, lips, whatever you caress, it'll up your intimacy levels. Intercourse, after all, is often about forging an emotional bond as well as a physical one. Why not let your hands help communicate that by showing her how much you love lavishing attention on her cute little mug?

Ride 'Em Cowgirl: Where Your Hands Can Roam When She's on Top

When women hop into the saddle, watch out: Study after study shows that women can most easily reach orgasm this way, and no wonder. Being in charge of the motion and angle of entry greatly increases the odds she'll have it just how she likes it. What's more, in this position, her partner's hands are wonderfully free to cause even more mischief. While the top gal may have a tougher time using her hands since she may be using her arms for support, she can still swing some pretty scorching moves if she makes a few tiny adjustments. Here are some ideas to get you yelling *yee-haw* in no time.

ROW HER BOAT

Must be done from the bottom

While one of the big benefits of being on top is that it gives women good clitoral stimulation, the bottom partner can give her even *more* by placing his thumbs to each side of this supersensitive nub. Then start paddling your thumbs by pressing one then the other alternately into the flesh. Start slow with one thumb pad press per second, and if that goes well, you can kick things up to about five per second. Let her be the captain and tell you what pressure and speed feels best, or just follow her lead. If she's going slow, do the same; once she picks up the pace, let your thumbs do the same.

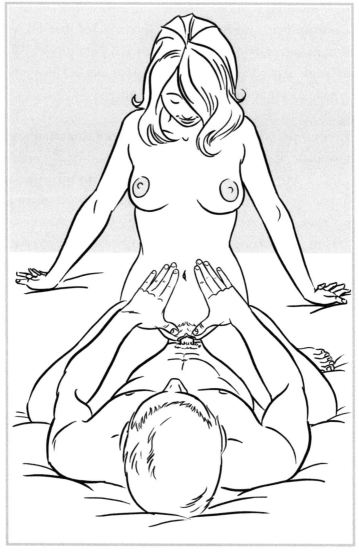

ROW HER BOAT

JUMP-START THE SACRUM (HER)

Must be done from the bottom

When she's moving slowly or taking a break and remaining stationary, reach around her waist and place your hands on her sacrum, a bone in the lower back that's hooked up straight to the genitals via the sacral nerve. To activate this stimulating connection, drum your fingers against it or press down on the sacrum. This will also get her clitoris rubbing even more snugly up against you, creating additional arousal points.

BOSOM BUDDIES

Must be done from the bottom

In woman-on-top lovemaking, her breasts all but beg to be fondled. Try letting your hands drift over her Grand Tetons barely touching them, or spread your five fingers over each breast and slowly draw your fingers in toward the nipple. While these techniques are best tried when she's moving slowly or not moving at all, once she speeds up and nears her orgasmic finale, consider giving her nips a playful pinch or tug to top things off.

HOLDING THE REINS

Must be done from on top

Ladies, now it's *your* turn to drive your guy crazy. Leaning back a bit (you can place a palm on his thigh for support), reach behind and caress his testicles while you ride him into the sunset. When you feel he might be about to blow, stop all movement and gently pull the testicles away from his body for a few seconds. The testicles hunch up right before ejaculation, and by pulling them away from his body, you delay his finale until you decide you're done with him.

TAMING THE BULL

Must be done from on top

If you want a little more romance mixed in with all that hedonistic humping, pour some massage oil on the center of the bottom partner's chest and massage the area in circles. This will stir up his sentimental side (in his heart) and cause him to subconsciously associate those warm and fuzzy feelings with all that randy rubbing down below. In effect, you're psychologically conditioning him to see sex as an extremely intimate experience. For further fireworks, move your hips in circles rather than just back and forth, which will get your genitals rubbing up against each other in a whole new array of angles you'll both enjoy.

RIDE 'EM COWGIRL IN REVERSE

Most easily done from on top

In this twist on the classic position, the woman turns around so that she's facing her partner's feet. From there she can remain vertical or lean back so she's lying on his chest before she starts gyrating. Unlike the traditional woman-on-top pose, this variation exposes the woman's clitoris to all kinds of hands-on activities. If you're on top, reach down (or around her body if you're the bottom partner and you can reach) and try rubbing the flat of your finger along the clitoris, tapping the bud with a fingertip, drumming your fingers on the mons pubis, or cupping the vulva and jiggling.

THE BIG TOE BONANZA

Must be done from on top

For this technique the woman again rides her guy in reverse so she's facing his feet. Only this time she leans forward and grabs each of his big toes before she starts moving her hips. You may recall from chap-

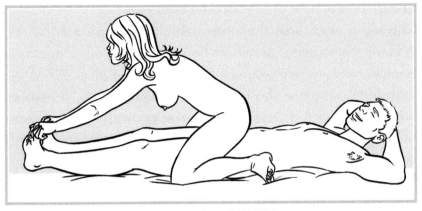

THE BIG TOE BONANZA

ter 4 that the big toe contains a ton of reflexology points that are linked to various parts of the body, including the pituitary gland, which is responsible for hormone production. This means that by squeezing the big toes you're firing up a whole lot more than just his feet. If he's loving it, consider disengaging from intercourse for a spell, scooting down, and sucking on those little piggies for extra points.

THE BIG TOE/BACK DOOR COMBO
Requires both partners' participation

Doing The Big Toe Bonanza presents the bottom partner with a whole new opportunity staring him straight in the face: his partner's butt. While the woman is moving slowly or remaining still, reach down and try spreading the cheeks apart, then together, one up one down then vice versa, or placing your thumbs to the sides of the anus and spreading them apart, then diagonally, then up and down. If she's up for more, massage circles along the sides of the rectum or massage her G-spot through the rectum.

Doing It Doggy-Style: Handy Tricks for Extra Kicks

This highly erotic, animalistic pose can fuel some extremely hot sex. And whether the guy stationed out back is kneeling or standing on the floor, his hands are free to do all sorts of scintillating things. While typically front partners are busy propping themselves up on all fours, by leaning forward on one shoulder, they, too, can reach for an assortment of hot spots. Here are some ideas to get you both panting in pleasure.

C-SPOT RUN

Must be done from the back

This one's simple: The guy reaches around the woman and stimulates her clitoris with his hands. When you first get going, start with something light, like rubbing the flat of your finger along her love button. Once things heat up, take the shaft of her clitoris between thumb and forefinger and stroke up and down. Once you two are on the brink of your finale, cup the entire vulva in your hand and shake. Since this trio of techniques builds in intensity, it should help keep you both on the same level arousal-wise and might even get you two reaching your peaks simultaneously.

G-SPOT RUN

Must be done from the back

If there's room, the guy can position his hand under his penis and insert a finger into the vagina during intercourse so that he can reach her G-spot—the extra-sensitive area located along the front wall around one to three inches in. To stimulate this erogenous zone, crook your finger in a come-hither motion, which would mean you're wiggling toward the floor. While thrusting may be compro-

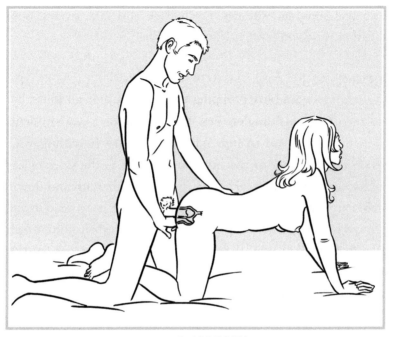

G-SPOT RUN

mised a bit and may need to proceed at a slower pace, the growls of enthusiasm you may soon hear will more than make up for this small inconvenience. If you find you can't insert a finger while your penis is inside her vagina, take a break from intercourse entirely to stimulate her G-spot before diving back in.

C-SPOT/G-SPOT COMBO
Can be done from the back or by both partners
For this move, the man slows down thrusting then uses *both* hands, combining G-spot Run with C-spot Run. Or, if the woman leans

down on one shoulder, she can reach back and take over C-spot duties. Either way, you'll be doubling her fun.

THE CAN CAN

Must be done from the back

As most men have probably noticed, in this position a woman's rear end is all but served up to him on a platter. Try twiddling your thumbs on the opening, or placing your thumbs to the sides of her anus and spreading them apart, then diagonally, then up and down. And if she's up for more in-depth exploration, feel free to head in and massage circles along the sides of the rectum or crook your finger along the front wall around three inches in to stimulate her G-spot. Given that heading in the back door can be a delicate process, you may want to remain stationary while easing your way in, and only resume intercourse once your partner is ready.

BACK FOR MORE

Must be done from the back

To give doggy-style sex a more sensual vibe, guys can give their partner a back and shoulder massage while going at it. Using massage oil, try pressing the heels of your palms up along the sides of her spine, fan out, then loop your way back down. Or you might want to form a U with your hand and push it up the sides of her spine. It also feels good to then cross your thumbs, spread your fingers, then glide your hands from her sacrum to the nape of her neck. All of these moves are easy to incorporate from the beginning to the end of intercourse. Women are suckers for men who remember that sex isn't just about the genitals, so this technique is true to its name: She'll be back for more in no time.

ME TARZAN, YOU JANE

Must be done from the back

If you want to add gasoline to the fire and transition to a true call of the wild carnal encounter, reach forward, hold the hair near the nape of her neck (the larger the chunk, the better), and gently pull toward you. Not only will this stimulate her scalp, it will most likely get her arching her back, allowing you to penetrate even deeper. This technique almost begs for some fast, intense thrusting action from one or both partners, although remember that you should never push past your partner's comfort zone.

THE JEWEL THIEF

Must be done from the front

In the doggy-style position a man's testicles are also ripe for the petting. If you're in front and want to reach them, lean your weight on one shoulder and extend an arm back between your thighs and his. From there you can try stroking the testicles with your fingertips or fingernails throughout intercourse, or gently pinch the seam between his testicles and pull on it occasionally. If he's close to Kingdom Come and you want to put ejaculation on hold, tell him to stop thrusting for a moment then use your thumb and forefinger to encircle the base of his testicles and pull them away from his body. While the guy out back typically thinks he's the alpha male in this position, this will show him you're not exactly taking it lying down, now are you?

PRESSING THE FLESH

Must be done from the front

As with The Jewel Thief, lean on one shoulder and reach back between your legs and his, only this time aim for his perineum, the patch of skin between his testicles and anus that is highly sensitive due to the prostate gland that lies underneath. To turn it on, press up and jiggle your hand. If your partner hums or moans while you're doing it, this will send pleasurable vibrations shooting up from his prostate to his throat and get his entire torso humming (for more details, turn to Good Vibes in chapter 6).

Sex Side-by-Side: How Your Hands Can Make It Sizzle

The perfect position for low-key, languid lovemaking, side-by-side sex comes with some unique perks. First off, couples can't easily engage in their usual high-impact thrusting—and that's a good thing, since you are forced to slow down and savor each sensation. Second, *both* sets of hands (yours and your partner's) are free to make mischief. Here's some territory you should consider covering.

THE SILVER SPOON

Can be performed by either partner

If you're spooning (where one partner's back lies snug against the other's belly), the woman's clitoris is free and clear to be approached by the partner out back. Reach around her body and try rubbing the flat of your finger along the clitoris or tapping on the bud with a fingertip. Or, if the woman reaches down and tends to her own privates, your hands can wander elsewhere. Consider letting your hands drift over her breasts barely touching them, or caressing her nipples alternately with your nails and your palm. Since these techniques require some finesse, combine them with a slow thrusting motion or remain completely stationary, focusing on your partner's pleasure. The woman can also squeeze her pubococcygeal (or PC) muscle (the one she uses to stop urinating) to provide additional stimulation.

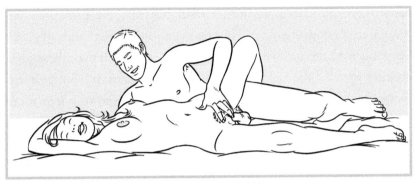

THE SILVER SPOON

TENDING TO THE FIELDS

Can be performed by either partner

During spooning, a woman's clitoris isn't the only hot spot calling out for attention; the furry mound of her mons pubis is also fully exposed. Reaching around her body, try undulating your hand on the area, or drumming your fingers on the top. You may also want to cup the mons and shake it back and forth to get some passion rumbling. Granted, moving your hips and your hands at the same time will require some coordination, but take it slow or alternate back and forth between handiwork and hip work and there will be plenty of feel-good vibes to go around.

IN THE GROOVE

Can be performed by either partner

Couples can also have sex side by side facing each other, which offers plenty of eye contact that intimacy gourmands will adore. While thrusting and penetration can be tough to accomplish in this position, these obstacles can open doors to *new* possibilities in the pleasure department. For example, rather than inserting the penis *into* the vagina, reach down between your bodies and use your hands to guide his penis into the groove between the inner labia. Then, through a rocking motion, rub his penis along this groove from front to back. Not only will this stimulate the extra-sensitive head of his penis; it will also hit many of *your* hot spots located along this sexy strip, including the clitoris, U-spot, and vagina. This move is proof positive that penetration doesn't have to happen for sex to feel fabulous, although if he's dying for a dip, the next time he slides back toward the vagina, let him keep going.

THE RATTLESNAKE

Can be performed by either partner

This technique is a tantalizing time-out from intercourse and easily follows from In the Groove. When the head of the penis is against the clitoris, reach down between your bodies, hold the penis by the base, and give it a shake. This will stimulate both the clitoris and the head of the penis, and that should make you both very, very happy.

SHAKE IT UP, BABY! SEX ADVENTURES FOR TRULY DARING DUOS

Now that you've got a handle on all the ways you can use your hands during your usual mattress maneuvers, let's explore beyond that. Whether you're curious to road-test sex toys, try a lovemaking position that's outside the norm, or dabble in a little light bondage or S&M, your hands can help in all these areas, too. So the next time you and your partner are feeling extra frisky, peruse this list for something that'll catch your fancy and fire things up in a whole new way.

SEX STANDING UP

There's something undeniably hot about two people who are just so into each other that they don't even bother to head to bed, much less find a flat surface, to stage their lovemaking. That said, having sex while standing is tricky for most couples due to issues of height, weight, and plain old gravity. But, as usual, you can turn to your hands for a little assistance. For one, we're assuming you two can most likely make it over to a wall, at which point the man can lift a woman up by her butt and lean her torso against the wall so he doesn't have to hoist her full mass midair. Second, if the woman can find something to grab onto, she can help to further lighten the load. One prime (and very passionate) example of this is in the movie *The Last Seduction,* where actress Linda Fiorentino ravishes Peter Berg against a chain link fence by clinging to it with her hands. While you might not have a fence available for such a feat (at least not in a private enough area), keep an eye out for other options around your home and you may be surprised what turns up. A very sturdy wall-mounted coat rack is one possibility; floor-to-ceiling built-in bookcases are another option as long as they're sturdy and won't fall on top of you. Or you can simulate standing-up sex by having the man stand at the edge of the bed facing out and having the woman prop her feet on the mattress and put her arms around the guy's shoulders. (*Warning:* Swinging from a shower curtain or chandelier, while tempting, is not a good idea.)

THE YAB YUM

In this classic Tantric pose, both the man and the woman are seated facing each other, with the woman's legs draped over his. This position is depicted in many ancient paintings and sculptures, and for good reason: It's a phenomenal way to connect with your partner and

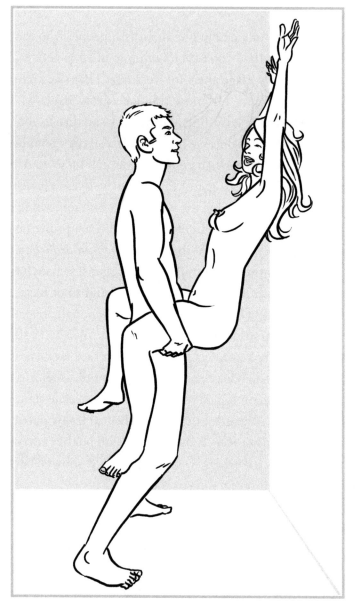

SEX STANDING UP

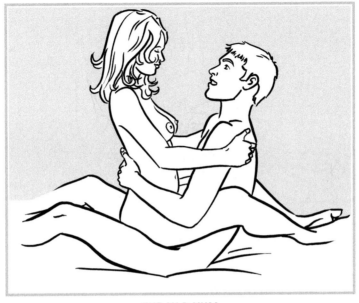

THE YAB YUM

exchange energy. Your thrusting abilities may be limited to more of a rocking motion, but that just opens doors for building arousal in other ways—and since all four hands are free, there's a lot you can do. Swap face, scalp, or back massages while you kiss and gaze into each other's eyes. If you're in the mood for some truly soul-moving sex, this may be the way.

THE SUMERIAN SQUAT

According to legend this was the signature sex position of Inanna, the ancient Mesopotamian goddess of sexual love, fertility, and war. Try it and you'll find it definitely has a bit of an "I am woman, hear me roar" allure. Not surprisingly, the woman is on top and the man

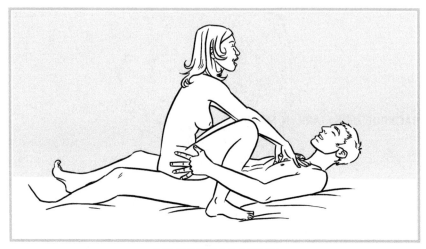

THE SUMERIAN SQUAT

below; only rather than resting on her knees, the woman places the soles of her feet flat on the bed then squats onto his penis. One thing you'll quickly notice about this position is that it requires very strong thigh muscles, but your guy's hands can be a lifesaver—just have him place his hands on your cute derrière and help move you up and down. Meanwhile you can place your hands on his chest for extra balance, and can massage his pecs or give his nipples a playful tug. If you lean forward farther, you can wrap your hands around his neck or shoulders and massage the area.

BREAST SEX

Massage oil a must

If your boobs are sized just right you can lather them up with massage oil then squeeze them together. Your man can then straddle your stomach and thrust into the sexy crevice between them. From the guy's viewpoint, this looks—and feels—sublime. For added pleasure, you can massage your breasts in circles or squeeze them together then release them. Plus he can reach back and start pushing your below-the-belt buttons to return the favor.

BACKRUB À LA MARILYN MONROE

Granted, giving your partner a back massage might not seem like a very racy way to spend the evening. But that's only because you've never tried Marilyn's version, which, rumor has it, prompted her to coyly mention, "I think I made his back feel better," after one of her "private meetings" with President John F. Kennedy. Here's how you can replicate her alleged sexy success: Lie your guy down and straddle his butt—ideally naked—and give him a sensual rubdown. Once he is relaxed, lean forward and whisper, "Wanna help make me come? Then lie very, very still . . ." Situating your mons pubis so it is pressing directly against his tailbone, start rocking your hips in small circles, finding which motion hits your personal sweet spot. Then ride him to your peak. Meanwhile you can continue massaging his back and whispering that you're getting hotter and hotter, closer and closer . . . Still think back massages are on the tame side? We didn't think so.

Sex Toy Tricks

Sex toys are like Disneyworld for your genitals, delivering never-before-felt thrills with the help of a little battery power (or an electrical outlet). And yet no matter how many types of good, good vibrations you've sampled over the years, odds are you haven't tried this trick, which gets your hands doing a whole lot more than just holding that gadget in the right spot. Try placing the sex toy in the palm of your hand and closing your fingers around it, or just pressing down on it with your thumb to hold it in place (ideally it should be a small sex toy). Turn the toy on and your whole hand should shake—which means that your fingers can now deliver the same buzz-worthy sensations as the toy itself.

This simple act of transference can be an incredible boon during sex, since you can now serve up the speed and power of a sex toy with more of a human touch. So consider keeping a sex toy cupped in your palm when doing any assortment of the techniques described in this book. In particular, try it with Good Vibes (a technique from chapter 6 where you press your fist—which is now holding a sex toy—into the guy's perineum) or The Shimmy (a technique from chapter 8 where you gently hold her inner labia, only in this instance you let the sex toy's vibrations travel on up).

Talk Dirty to Me

Weaving in some X-rated conversation while your hands are wandering can make for an incredibly erotic experience. If you tend to get tongue-tied, here are a few pointers to get you started. First, you and your partner should have a discussion about exactly which words you find a turn-on and a turnoff. Some women, for example, might find it hot to hear someone call them a "slut"; others might totally detest the term. Likewise some men may prefer you call their equipment a "cock" rather than the diminutive-sounding "willy." Our point is that the very same lovemaking lingo can trigger completely different reactions based on whom you're talking to, so it can help to come to an agreement beforehand on which words you should use and which you should avoid.

Once you've got some hot vocabulary to work with and your hands start roaming, what next? Basically, there are three very easy ways to break the ice. The first and probably easiest is to merely ask your partner a question, such as "Do you want me to touch your [fill in the blank]?" or "Why don't you come over here and play with my [fill in the blank]?" The second way to get started is to describe something you're about to do ("Next I'm going to put my fingers in your [bleep]") or something you're currently doing ("Now my fingers are sliding inside your [bleep]"). Finally, you can ask your partner if he or she likes the results ("Do you like it when I [bleep] your [bleep]?").

Pretty much all of these explicit talk techniques can also be used during phone sex (and just think of how happy your partner would be to receive *that* call). So if one of you is on a business trip or you two are otherwise miles apart, pick up the phone (preferably at a time when you know your partner has some privacy) and say, "I wish you were here so I could throw you down on the bed and . . ." Or describe what you're doing to yourself, as in, "Now my hands are fondling my nipples, caressing my stomach, slipping under my pants . . ." Those are just a few of the many ways your handiwork can be combined with some sexy conversation. Go ahead and whisper, growl, or even shout your praises to add an audio element to lovemaking.

Breakin' Out the Blindfolds

Deny yourself the use of your peepers and all your other senses sharpen to compensate: hearing, smell, taste, and—most important—your sense of touch. So try tying a scarf over your partner's eyes before your hands start wandering. Whatever you're doing, ask your partner to tell you how it ranks on a scale of one (not so pleasurable) to ten (pleasurable beyond belief). This will help you both tune in to subtler nuances that turn you on. Afterward, switch so you're the one who is blindfolded and soaking up a rich new realm of sensations.

Tie Me Up, Tie Me Down

There's a whole culture and tons of literature devoted to the art of bondage, and since we're not experts in this area we would highly recommend that you look elsewhere for a deeper understanding of how to start experimenting safely. Still, what we *do* know is that you don't need handcuffs, rope, or restraints of any kind to begin, since your hands alone can do a pretty good job at simulating their effects. Playfully pin your partner's wrists over his or her head on the bed, or order your partner to sit on his or her hands and not move an inch. While your partner isn't *really* helpless in these scenarios, the feeling may well up just the same.

Once your partner's hands are "tied up" so to speak, then what? While pretty much anything you do will feel edgier because your partner is powerless to stop you, to truly take advantage of the situation, a little teasing is in order. Stroke around, but not on, your partner's choice spots. Bring your partner to the brink of orgasm then pull back, then build again. The results will drive your partner nuts, but that will only make the moment when you *do* deliver the goods all the more gratifying.

From Ow! to Wow! Turning Pain into Pleasure

For some people pain feels, well, painful. And yet for others pain feels absolutely fabulous, provided it's within the context of a sexual relationship where both partners are in on the game. Again, since S&M isn't our area of expertise, you'll want to turn elsewhere for in-depth instructions. Still, if you're interested in delivering just one or two playful swats just to kick things up a notch, we can certainly provide your hands with some pointers.

The secret to delivering slaps that feel pleasurable rather than painful is to cup your hand so you're hitting with less surface area and keep your hand relaxed while slapping. While the rump is your most obvious bull's-eye, the inner thighs, soles of the feet, chest/breasts, and even a woman's mons pubis are all respectable targets. Just be sure to steer clear of the kidneys (the area above the buttocks) and, of course, his family jewels. Start with light slaps and rub the area between smacks, which will cut down on the sting and create a more sensual vibe. If you up the intensity, gauge your partner's reaction closely. You can either focus on spanking and save sex for later, switch back and forth, or spank and shag simultaneously. For the last option, you'll find that doggy-style sex is ideal since your partner's rump is right in front of you, although you can also reach around during missionary or woman-on-top lovemaking to pat that posterior.

Lights, Camera, Action! How to Pull Off an Oscar-worthy Role-Playing Scenario

To many the prospect of role-playing feels ridiculous rather than arousing. Reserve judgment until you try it, though, and you may soon change your tune. Take on a new persona and suddenly you've got carte blanche to do or say things the "real" you wouldn't dream of. If, for example, you're usually a go-with-the-flow kinda gal, playing "the boss" to your partner's "employee" gives you permission to switch gears into ball-busting mode. Or if you're a guy who is usually calling the shots in bed, playing "patient" to your partner's "nurse" can snap you into subservience. And no, you don't need elaborate costumes or a script's worth of lines, just a quick discussion with your partner about the parameters is all that's needed to get things rolling. So, if you're up for an escape from your usual patterns, consider finding a role-playing plot you like and give it a go.

In the following paragraphs we have outlined a few scenarios you might want to try, as well as described how to pull them off. All require their own unique breed of handiwork, and each experience may be a hit on your arousal charts.

Doctor/patient: The patient makes an appointment claiming to be suffering from a mysterious ailment; the doctor (or nurse) performs a hands-on, hot 'n' heavy exam to pinpoint exactly where the patient's "ache" is coming from. You can perform a "breast exam" where you palpate the tissue or explore areas below the belt, closely gauging your partner's reaction and asking how it feels. Once your hands have found the spot that most needs your medical attention, go ahead and provide the cure. Orgasms, after all, are good for your health.

Stripper/client: The client purchases a lap dance and sits back to enjoy the show. The stripper starts gyrating, slowly peeling off layers of clothing, stroking, squeezing, and gently slapping his/her own hot spots—and the client's—along the way. To be an even bigger tease, establish a No Touching Allowed rule for clientele (although in this case maybe rules are meant to be broken?).

First date duo: Even if you two have been together for years, pretend you've only just met. Make out in the car or on your couch, but say you aren't willing to go all the way. By taking the intercourse card out of the equation, you bring your foreplay skills—largely conducted using your hands—to the forefront and are forced to get creative with all kinds of manual moves. While holding hands, trace a circle in your partner's palm with your thumb to steam things up. Or, if your hands are wandering under your "date's" shirt, caress the chest or, on a woman, brush your fingertips over the silky material of her bra. Let your hands snake up the inner thigh and caress over the undies . . . or under them.

Masseuse or masseur/client: The client books an appointment for a rubdown, describing exactly which areas are most "sore" and in need of a little TLC. The masseuse/masseur promises to work out *all* the kinks . . . and maybe even throw in a "happy ending" to boot.

CONCLUSION

If you began this book thinking *Honestly, how much of an asset can your hands really be in bed?*, we hope by now we have convinced you that if you give your hands a chance, they will surprise, astound, and amaze you and your partner. Try even just a few of the techniques in these pages and the proof will be palpable: In bed you'll hear more moaning, have deeper, longer-lasting, and more frequent orgasms, and suddenly find a zillion excuses to sneak off and do it again . . . and again. Your hands can lift your sex life to incredible heights because that's what they're *designed* to do. What's more, if you take the time to really look at your lover's body as well as your own, you will realize that there is no better, more beautiful canvas on which your hands can work their magic.

There are two things above all else that we hope you take away from this book. The first is that it doesn't really matter whether you can perform these techniques on your partner to a tee. All that really matters is that you two touch, period, as often as possible, in bed and out of bed. Hold hands during movies. Give him a hug when you scoot past him in the kitchen. And if she's had a hard day at work, treat her to a shoulder rub. These tiny gestures of affection will keep the passion alive between you so that by the time you do head to bed, all kinds of cool, crazy things may happen.

The second thing we hope you take away from this book is this: that as nice as it feels to kick back and get pampered by someone who cares about you, *giving* pleasure can be even more satisfying than receiving it. In today's sexual landscape, that may sound as corny as the pickup lines being bandied about in bars. But it's true. And *giving* is what your hands do best. They stick money into the March of Dimes canister, put food on the table come dinnertime, and even type sweet e-mails like "Had an amazing time last night—how about a repeat on Friday?"

Using your hands to their full potential means always keeping an eye out for the good they can accomplish. Do that and you're well on your way to a better relationship, and a better sex life.

The larger heart, the kindlier hand!

—ALFRED, LORD TENNYSON

ACKNOWLEDGMENTS

Writing this book has been an amazing experience that would have never happened without the guidance of the following people:

First and foremost, a huge thank you goes to Douglas Stewart, our agent at Sterling Lord Literistic, Inc., whose enthusiasm and unflappable attitude made our first foray into book publishing a joy from beginning to end.

Warmest thanks also go to our mentors and colleagues Joseph Kramer, Ph.D. and Kenneth Ray Stubbs. Their pioneering work in the field of sexological bodywork and erotic massage has proven invaluable for this field. They've taught us so much over the years and are incredible friends we feel blessed to know.

Thank you to Scott D. Bahlmann for additional uncircumcised techniques, Jeffrey Raymond for helping us with new techniques and for many days of being a guinea pig for practice (we know you didn't mind), Destin Gerek for an interesting night of photographs for the illustrations in this book, and to Jim Perry for your love and support—you really are family to us.

Special and heartfelt thanks to Ian Ferguson, whose support helped dreams come true, and to Kurtis Bliss and Lawrence Lanoff, two fellow visionaries and artists who have supported this project in numerous, uncountable ways. To all people everywhere living a life of embodiment and peaceful sexual exploration, you are all pioneers; our gratitude goes out with full force to each of you.

APPENDIX

This book is a small glimpse of all that we have to offer. We teach all over the United States and abroad; for a complete schedule of workshops and lectures or for more information please visit our Web site at www.touchingdeeply.com.

To purchase Jon and Jaiya's DVDs and sign up for their free newsletter, go to www.newworldsexeducation.com.

To contact Jaiya and find out more information about her, go to www.missjaiya.com.

For more information about Jon or to contact him, go to www.tantrabodies.com.

You can watch the techniques in this book in the comfort of your own home through streaming video at www.redhottouch.tv.

You can enjoy streaming video demonstrations of many of the pleasurable teachings in this book at the New School of Erotic Touch. This school is the best online resource to help you learn vulva, penis, and anal massage. Go to www.eroticmassage.com.

If you are considering becoming a teacher of erotic massage, we recommend that you earn a Sexological Bodywork certification through the Institute for Advanced Study of Human Sexuality. We learned a lot taking this professional, California-approved training. We sometimes coteach this course with Joseph Kramer, Ph.D. For more information, visit www.sexologicalbodywork.com.

Kenneth Ray Stubbs is a pioneer of erotic massage for couples and has contributed a body of books and DVDs on enhancing lovemaking. For more information about him or to view his works, visit www.secretgardenpublishing.com.

We have also extensively trained and practiced the Ipsalu Tantra Kriya Yoga path. For more information about Ipsalu Tantra and to view their workshop schedule, visit www.tantrabliss.com.

To buy condoms (including female condoms), go to www.undercovercondoms.com.

For a great selection of gloves that you can use during your massage and anal play (vinyl or nitrile), visit www.massagewarehouse.com.

For a full selection of sex toys and personal lubricants, go to www.goodvibes.com or www.toysinbabeland.com.

For homeopathic personal lubricants for those with sensitive skin or allergies, visit www.sympathical.com.

Coconut oil is our favorite massage oil and lube. We've tried many coconut oils, but not all are created equal. Here's where you can get our favorite: www.nutiva.com.

RECOMMENDED READING AND VIEWING

Chia, Mantak, and Douglas Abrams. *The Multi-orgasmic Man.* HarperCollins, 2002.

Chia, Mantak, Maneewan Chia, Douglas Abrams, and Rachel Carlton Abrams. *The Multi-Orgasmic Couple: Sexual Secrets Every Couple Should Know.* HarperOne, 2002.

Chia, Mantak, and William U. Wei. *Sexual Reflexology: Activating the Taoist Points of Love.* Destiny Books, 2003.

Chopra, M.D., Deepak. *Deepak Chopra: Kama Sutra.* Virgin Books, 2006.

Lai, Hsi. *The Sexual Teachings of the White Tigress: Secrets of the Female Taoist Masters.* Destiny Books, 2001.

Natale, Frank. *Mastering Alive Relationships.* T.N.I., 1990.

Saraswati, Sunyata, and Bodhi Avinasha. *The Jewel in the Lotus / The Tantric Path to Higher Consciousness.* Ipsalu Publishing, 2002.

Schulte, Christa. *Tantra for Women: A Guide for Lesbian, Bi, Hetero, and Solo Lovers.* Hunter House, 2005.

Stubbs, Kenneth Ray. *Erotic Massage: The Tantric Touch of Love.* Tarcher, 1999.

———. *Femme a Femme Erotic Massage.* (DVD) Secret Garden Publishing, 2007.

ABOUT THE AUTHORS

Jaiya and Jon Hanauer are certified sexological bodyworkers with certificates from the Institute for the Advanced Study of Human Sexuality in San Francisco. They are members of the Association for Sexual Energy Professionals (ASEP) and the Association for Certified Sexological Bodyworkers (ACSB). Together they have worked with hundreds of individuals and couples, conducting group workshops across the country and abroad on the power of touch. They are certified sex educators and Tantra teachers and practitioners; Jaiya has also been trained and practiced as a licensed massage therapist for close to ten years. Jaiya and Jon have been teaching together as a couple since 2001 and currently live in Los Angeles, where they have founded the New World Sex Education Production Company.

Julie Jeffries is a writer and editor living in Brooklyn, New York. She has worked for *Cosmopolitan*, *Maxim*, *Glamour*, *Redbook*, *Stuff*, Match.com, and other publications. She has covered a range of topics, including dating, relationships, sex, health, personal finance, news, and entertainment.